About the Author

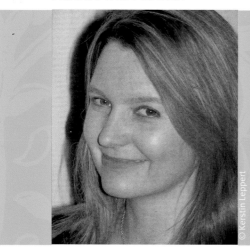

Kerstin Leppert has been a kundalini yoga teacher since 1994. She leads yoga classes as well as individual sessions for special problems and needs and is the editor of *Kundalini Yoga Journal* in Germany.

In addition to contributions to numerous professional journals and anthologies, she has published three volumes of poems and two novels. Her other books include *Das ErsteHilfebuch bei Liebeskummer* (The First Help Book for Lovesickness), *Nie mehr Stress* (No More Stress), *Nie mehr Schnupfen & Co* (No More Sniffles & Co.), and *Erfüller Sex mit Yoga* (Fulfilling Sex with Yoga).

Further information about her work is available at www.yogaundpilates .de and www.gedichte-pur.de.

Kerstin Leppert is married, has two children, and lives with her family in Hamburg, Germany.

IMPORTANT NOTE

The material in this book is intended to provide a review of information regarding a yoga plan designed to increase fertility. Every effort has been made to provide accurate and dependable information and the contents of this book have been compiled through professional research and in consultation with professionals. However, always consult your doctor or physical therapy practitioner before undertaking a new exercise regimen or doing any of the exercises or suggestions contained in this book, especially if you suffer from any chronic illness.

The author, publisher and its staff are not liable for any health or personal harm that may come to the reader, nor for their degree of success in following the methods prescribed herein. The author and publisher are not liable for any damage or injury or other adverse outcome of applying the information in this book in a program carried out independently or under the care of a licensed trainer or practitioner. Yoga can be practiced by everyone; however, it should be practiced mindfully, while paying close attention to your physical boundaries. If you have questions concerning the application of the information described in this book, consult a qualified and trained professional. In the case of acute illness, immediately stop your yoga practice.

Ordering
Trade bookstores in the U.S. and Canada please contact
Publishers Group West
1700 Fourth Street, Berkeley CA 94710
Phone: (800) 788-3123   Fax: (800) 351-5073

For bulk orders please contact
Special Sales
Hunter House Inc., PO Box 2914, Alameda CA 94501-0914
Phone: (510) 899-5041   Fax: (510) 865-4295
E-mail: sales@hunterhouse.com

Individuals can order our books by calling **(800) 266-5592**
or from our website at **www.hunterhouse.com**

fertility yoga

A Natural Approach to Conception

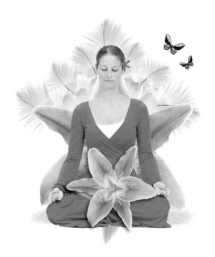

KERSTIN LEPPERT

Hunter House
PUBLISHERS

Hunter House Inc., Publishers
PO Box 2914
Alameda CA 94501-0914

Library of Congress Cataloging-in-Publication Data
Leppert, Kerstin, 1967-
[Fruchtbarkeitsyoga. English]
Fertility yoga : a natural approach to conception / Kerstin Leppert. — First edition.
       pages   cm
Includes bibliographical references and index.
ISBN 978-0-89793-648-4 (pbk.)   ISBN 978-0-89793-649-1 (ebook)
1. Meditation—Therapeutic use. 2. Kundalini—Therapeutic use. 3. Fertility, Human. I. Title.
RC489.M43L4713 2013
613.7'046—dc23   2012043826

Interior photos: p. 1 © lily, p. 3 © Stefan Balk, p. 6 © Jugulator, p. 16 © diez-artwork,
p. 21 and p. 140 © magann, p. 22 © vision images, p. 26 © Marco Mayer, p. 32 © EMrpize,
p. 35 © sarsmis, p. 44 © Angela, p. 51 © Sergey Peterman, p. 54 © angrylittledwarf,
p. 99 © Anette Linnea Rasmus, p. 102 © Christina Malsch, p. 112 and p. 123 © felinda,
p. 130 © Renate Flormann, p. 143 © PhotoSG, p. 154 © jundream, p. 148 © Andres Rodriguez,
p. 153 © Stephen Coburn—fotolia.com.

Project Credits

Cover Design: Peri Poloni-Gabriel	Administrative Assistant: Kimberly Kim
Book Production: John McKercher	Publicity Coordinator: Martha Scarpati
Translator: Leah Lowthorp	Special Sales Manager: Judy Hardin
Exercise Photos: Bert Harder, Kerstin Leppert	Rights Coordinator: Candace Groskreutz
Photo Models: Steven Beik,	Customer Service Manager:
Nicole Werner, Kerstin Leppert	Christina Sverdrup
Copy Editor: Kelley Blewster	Order Fulfillment: Washul Lakdhon
Indexer: Nancy D. Peterson	Administrator: Theresa Nelson
Managing Editor: Alexandra Mummery	Computer Support: Peter Eichelberger
Publisher's Assistant: Bronwyn Emery	Publisher: Kiran S. Rana

Printed and bound by Bang Printing, Brainerd, Minnesota
Manufactured in the United States of America

9 8 7 6 5 4 3 2 1   First U. S. Edition   13 14 15 16 17

Contents

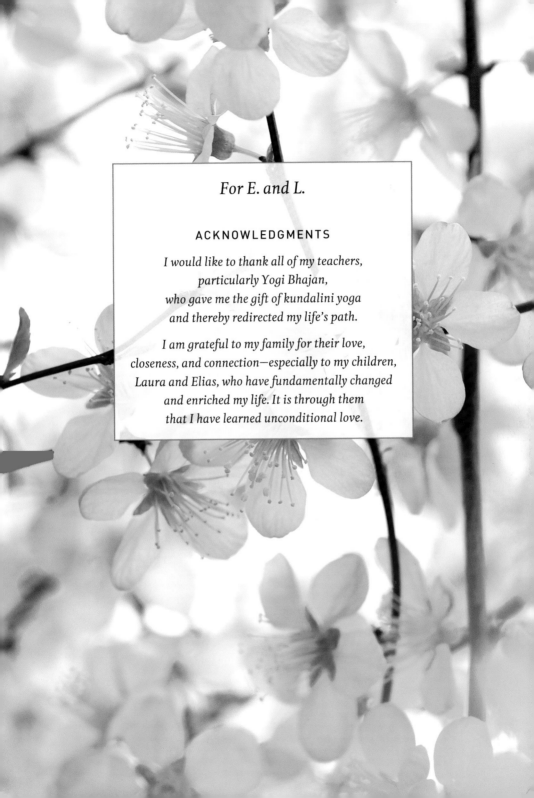

For E. and L.

ACKNOWLEDGMENTS

I would like to thank all of my teachers,
particularly Yogi Bhajan,
who gave me the gift of kundalini yoga
and thereby redirected my life's path.

I am grateful to my family for their love,
closeness, and connection—especially to my children,
Laura and Elias, who have fundamentally changed
and enriched my life. It is through them
that I have learned unconditional love.

Introduction

Dear Readers,

You have purchased this book because you have a strong desire to have a child. You've probably also decided to prepare for your pregnancy as much as you possibly can instead of letting things simply run their course. You most likely have already found your life partner, and together have chosen the optimal time to have a baby based on your career and life goals. You would like to prepare both your body and mind for the challenges of pregnancy and giving birth. The gentle but strengthening practice of fertility yoga is an ideal choice.

Fertility yoga is a system of body and breath exercises, meditations, visualizations, massage, and relaxation techniques. It is also a set of recommendations for how to lead your life, eat well, and heighten your consciousness. Fertility yoga as a whole seeks to support women and men who are on the path toward parenthood.

"We want a baby!" That sounds so simple, and for some it is. Some women get pregnant without much effort and also seem to go through the birthing process without any difficulty. For others, however, it is a longer and more-arduous journey from the point of wanting a child to the reality of actually having one. Despite all biological and medical explanations, the act of conceiving a baby is a miracle. It is unpredictable, even mystical. Yoga teaches that children are the ones who seek out their parents, not vice versa. You cannot expect that as soon as you stop using your regular method of birth control you will immediately get pregnant. Even though many people know of couples who were able to get pregnant easily, or have friends who have had unwanted pregnancies, such cases aren't necessarily the rule.

This book is for couples who have long wished for a child, a wish that for whatever reason has yet to be fulfilled. Perhaps you've passed the peak of fertility, which for women is in their mid-twenties and for men in their early forties. Perhaps you are a woman who has an irregular menstrual cycle. Perhaps you are worried about the root cause of your previous failed attempts to conceive and are contemplating medical intervention. Fertility yoga can help in all of these situations.

It encourages you to let go of your need for control and prepares both your body and mind for conception. The practice of fertility yoga can also be a meaningful supplement to fertility treatments.

One of the tenets of yoga is that life energy follows thought. Yoga can help to both stimulate and heighten fertility by increasing blood flow to reproductive organs and glands through movement and breath exercises. Men, who often have issues with fertility, can also benefit from these practices. The regular practice of yoga strengthens perception and bodily awareness, and helps you "get out of your head and into your gut or core." It can also help to alleviate other issues, such as PMS or painful periods. Moreover, it stimulates a woman's ovaries and optimizes her body's ability to conceive.

Fertility yoga works on more than just a physical level. Yoga is first and foremost a spiritual practice that helps us better manage life's challenges. Trying to get pregnant, with all of its accompanying hopes, worries, and fears, can be a challenging time for your nerves, relationships, and self-confidence. Those who practice yoga are giving themselves a gift—one that strengthens their sense of optimism, self-confidence, and serenity.

I wish you a satisfying and fulfilling journey!

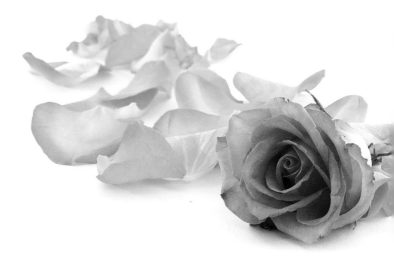

CHAPTER 1

HOW YOGA CAN HELP YOU CONCEIVE

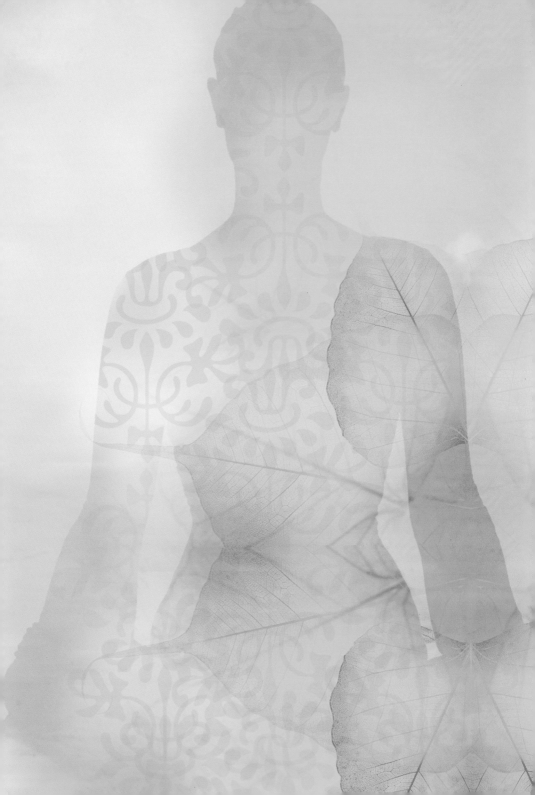

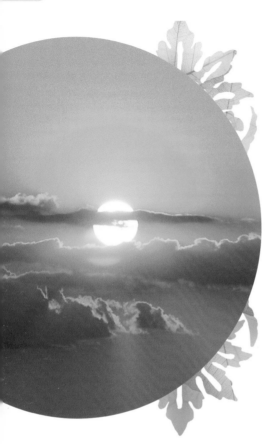

Fertility and the Menstrual Cycle

Beginning with a disclaimer that this is not medical advice, let us first take a brief look at the menstrual cycle. The average menstrual cycle is twenty-eight days long, with an actual range of twenty-one to thirty-five days. A woman is only fertile for three to five of those days. We will begin our count on the first day of the menstrual flow. The first phase, of varying duration, is the follicle- or egg-maturation phase. Next comes the luteal phase, or secretory phase, which lasts between twelve and fourteen days. Ovulation occurs between those two phases. The egg itself is only capable of being fertilized during a period of approximately twelve to eighteen hours. However, because sperm are able to survive for three to five days under "good" cervical conditions, the fertility window extends over several days.

Many women think they ovulate in the middle of their menstrual cycles. This is only true for women who have the standard twenty-eight-day cycle. In actuality, ovulation occurs twelve to fourteen days before the start of the menstrual flow. So a woman with a thirty-three-day cycle will ovulate on or around day nineteen, and a woman with a twenty-four-day cycle will ovulate on or around day ten. The fertility window closes when ovulation occurs, and conception becomes impossible for the rest of that particular menstrual cycle.

Research has shown that even if couples have intercourse during the woman's fertility window, the probability of becoming pregnant is only around 25 percent; on the day after ovulation this number falls below 1 percent.

For this reason, it is important for women to be aware of the rhythm of their own menstrual cycles.

Keep track of your cycle over several months. Pick out your longest and shortest cycles, and count back eighteen days to determine when your window of fertility usually opens. If, for example, your longest cycle was twenty-eight days and your shortest was twenty-two days, then your fertile period starts somewhere between day four and day ten of your cycle, and ovulation occurs somewhere between day eight and day fourteen. Your total window of fertility would thus begin on day four and end on day fourteen.

This means that women with very short cycles could be fertile during their actual menstrual flow. For women with longer cycles the fertile period gets pushed farther back, and for women with inconsistent cycles the possible window of fertility becomes quite large. To gain a more precise idea of your individual fertility, you can measure your temperature in the morning before getting out of bed to determine the end of your current fertile period. Start measuring your temperature every morning, and as soon as you observe a temperature increase of between 0.7 and 1.4 degrees Fahrenheit, you will know that you have ovulated in the last twelve to twenty-four hours. This knowledge can be used to determine your fertile period for your next cycle. You can also pay close attention to changes in your cervical mucus and your libido. This method requires a delicate system of self-observation that can be perfected with practice. Yoga helps you sharpen your sensitivity and awareness of your body. Cervical mucus varies from being dry or absent before the start of your menstrual flow, to cloudy and sticky before ovulation, to clear and slippery during ovulation. Around the time of ovulation many women feel a heightened sensuality and an increased desire to have sex with their partners. This makes complete sense from a biological standpoint: Nature wants you to reproduce by having sexual intercourse when you are most fertile. However, if you have been using hormonal birth control methods for a long time, it could take a while for your body to regain its natural rhythm.

If Pregnancy Eludes You

In earlier times, most women gave birth to their children at a young age. Even in the 1960s many women had already given birth to several children by their mid-twenties. In the last fifty years the average age of a woman at first birth has continued to climb in industrialized nations, and nowadays it is nearing thirty. When I gave birth to my daughter in 1993 at age twenty-five, I was the exception among my girlfriends, most of whom had not even begun to think about having children. In those days I used natural methods of birth control—though admittedly without being aware of my own, short menstrual cycle. My daughter was conceived on what I thought was a "safe" day, the fourth day of my cycle.

Most couples today follow a three-stage model: first, school and job training or college; second, a few years spent working; and third, searching for a partner and starting a family. According to current estimates, around 70 percent of pregnancies today are planned. After spending the greater part of

their most fertile years successfully avoiding pregnancy, many women stop taking the birth control pill and expect to get pregnant right away. For the majority of these women pregnancy occurs somewhere in their next twelve menstrual cycles. However, about ten or twenty percent of women still find themselves waiting for the blue line to appear on their pregnancy tests a full year later, and can often become increasingly disheartened. This constitutes a fertility problem, or infertility, meaning that no pregnancy has occurred after a full year of unprotected sexual intercourse. Statistically, the cause of infertility is attributed equally to the female and male partners, and sometimes, though less so, to both. Often there is no medical condition preventing pregnancy, which is called idiopathic infertility. Sometimes the problem is unknown or unidentifiable. Everything is still possible, but how are you supposed to pass the time when your biological clock keeps ticking louder and louder, and your desire to have a child starts to overwhelm you?

Increasing age does in fact make having a baby more difficult, because a woman's egg cells age as she ages. Baby girls are born with all of their eggs already fully formed in their ovaries. Beginning at puberty the eggs mature one by one each month and get shed with menstruation when they remain unfertilized. A woman's greatest years of fertility, between ages eighteen and twenty-four, are nowadays often behind her before she even starts to think about having children. This can cause a number of problems. "Older" eggs often have chromosomal issues that *decrease* their chance of being fertilized and *increase* their chance of being miscarried even if fertilized successfully. Ongoing, unresolved pelvic infections can lead to blockage of the fallopian tubes. If a woman suffers from endometriosis, or has had surgery on her ovaries, her chances of becoming pregnant can also decrease. There are a number of other medical reasons, for both men and women alike, that can make conceiving a child difficult. The main focus of this book, however, is not upon purely medical intervention methods. Instead, this book offers you advice on how to get in tune with your body and through the power of fertility yoga, increase your chances of having a baby.

How Stress Reduces Fertility

We are all expected to live in a never-ending cycle of stress and relaxation, to push ourselves past our limits, and to master every challenging situation we encounter. Nevertheless, only a few would find a life of relaxation spent perpetually lying in a hammock truly satisfying. As tempting as it sounds, most people would quickly grow bored with such a life. Many people feel overwhelmed by the pressures placed upon them, whether from their professional lives, their private lives, or even their recreational activities. It is beyond the scope of this book to get into an extended discussion about whether people should relax more or work harder. Suffice to say that the inner and outer pressures that affect us, both consciously and unconsciously, set in motion a complicated process that, left unchecked, can eventually lead to a state of chronic stress. Long-term sources of stress may include, for example, financial problems, an unsatisfying professional life, family worries, an absence of meaningful social connections, and an unfulfilling love life.

Stress is a subjective experience that is perceived and handled differently by each person. Some are more resistant to it than others. The roots of stress often lie in childhood or in one's biological constitution; some people who are naturally action-oriented and self-confident tend to stress out less than others. The pace of our world is growing faster, more hectic, and more stimulating, and our archaic nervous system can't always hold up. As a result many people seek out things that provide them respite, such as relaxation techniques. In my experience stress is usually the biggest motivation for why people start taking a yoga class. Most people who come to me seek to gain the ability to simply deactivate and let go.

Stress affects your thoughts, feelings, actions, and bodily functions. It also negatively influences fertility. It doesn't matter if it is positive stress, so-called eustress, or negative stress, also known as distress. Male and female reproductive organs don't operate independently from the rest of the body; fertility is controlled by hormones secreted by the endocrine system. The pituitary gland plays a central role in this as the organ that controls the whole process. Yogis maintain that it is the seat of the third eye (sixth chakra).

The pituitary gland is connected to the hypothalamus, a small but important part of the brain that controls the autonomic nervous system. The autonomic system regulates body temperature, heartbeat, blood pressure, absorption of food and water, sleep, and sexual and reproductive behavior. The pituitary gland therefore connects bodily and mental processes with each other. Feelings determine thoughts and relay information that is then translated by the body into physical reactions.

In the case of chronic stress, the body defends itself by drawing resources away from certain functions such as fertility that are not vital for survival. Symptoms of stress-induced infertility can include an irregular menstrual cycle, absent or excessive menstrual bleeding, fluctuating hormones, decreased sperm quality, yeast infections, or an inflamed prostate. Reproductive medicine has long debated the connection between body and mind, largely treating the body as a machine, but nowadays even more-orthodox doctors have increasingly arrived at the conclusion that stress and psychological problems like depression can negatively affect both the maturation of egg cells and the production and development of sperm.

Functional and Idiopathic Infertility

The underlying causes for difficulties in conceiving can lie on either a functional or idiopathic level. Functional infertility is related to the workings of the body itself. It is measurable, and in many cases able to sort itself out on its own. It has both physical and psychological causes. It is often a result of a female hormonal imbalance, such as too little or too much follicle-stimulating hormone (FSH) or luteinizing hormone (LH) in the blood, which can lead to a lack of ovulation, or fluctuating prolactin and thyroid hormone levels, which also restrict fertility. Primary or secondary amenorrhea, when menstruation fails to occur at puberty or occurs and then ceases later in life, can often have psychological roots. Psychological stress in men can also cause decreased sperm quality.

Idiopathic infertility, also known as unexplained infertility, is caused by neither physical nor hormonal issues. The male partner's sperm quality can be high and the female partner can be free of any fertility issues, but the couple still doesn't get pregnant. This situation is often the most agonizing for a couple, because it seems as if everything is and should be functioning perfectly. Feelings of failure, guilt, and inferiority can result, as well as deeper soul searching and a reevaluation of one's life. A long-held, deep-seated desire to have children can feel especially burdensome and may lead to a vicious circle that can only be broken by consciously learning to let go of these regrets.

The Need for Control and Letting Go

A lot of couples believe, either consciously or unconsciously, that it is possible to plan a pregnancy. This causes them to apply the same meticulousness they used earlier to avoid pregnancy to getting pregnant. Some couples grow impatient shortly after their first attempts to get pregnant, quickly seeking out medical advice and intervention. People who are driven and goal oriented, and who have accomplished much in life through diligence, determination, and planning, may expect immediate success when applying these same methods to getting pregnant. Accustomed to managing their lives through brain power, they fail to take into account that the body has its own wisdom and often fights back the more one tries to control it. If pregnancy does not occur right away, such individuals may be vulnerable to becoming caught in a never-ending cycle of stress: The more a pregnancy is forced, the longer it remains unsuccessful, and the more determinedly a couple researches its possible causes and visits fertility clinics that focus on purely technical answers.

Results-oriented thinking can be seen in the word choice couples often employ: "Let's make a baby," or "Let's have a baby." Conceiving a child, however, is an act of devotion, of letting go, and of simply being ready. It is often difficult for action-oriented individuals to simply let go and let conception occur in its own time. Instead, they try to control

their bodies through all means available, so that it "finally works." When the couple eventually does get pregnant, they start to consult a new set of experts to ensure that the pregnancy runs smoothly and a healthy child is born.

The belief that it is possible to fully control the creation of a new life, however, is a misconception. Especially in the cases of functional and idiopathic infertility, it often seems as if your body is rebelling against your mental demands upon it to conceive a child.

Instead of respecting and loving your body, your mind tries to force the body to obey its will by getting pregnant. Some people's bodies start to withdraw the more the mind tries to control them, through an increasingly irregular menstrual cycle that makes the hormones go haywire or through decreased sperm quality.

There have even been studies showing that women who were trying to get pregnant actually took longer to accomplish their goal than women who weren't trying to control the process. A goal-oriented approach might work to guarantee professional success, but it is much less effective in controlling organic processes such as the functioning of your own body.

What can help you to move away from a need for control, toward an ability to let go and let things simply take their course? For one, realizing that it doesn't help to obsessively measure your body temperature, observe the changes in your cervical mucus, or have your partner's sperm quality constantly assessed. On the other hand, beginning the bodily practice of yoga will help you rediscover your senses and bodily awareness. And yoga can do so much more: It quiets the bustling train of thought and stills the busy mind—at least for as long as it takes to complete one breath.

Psychological Barriers

There can be many reasons why a person's psyche would protect their body from being dominated by the mind, thus preventing a pregnancy. Here I list only a few possible reasons. First, underlying

difficulties could be encumbering a couple's relationship, which can begin when the desire for having a child is not expressed equally by both partners. Often one partner, usually the woman, will feel a more urgent desire to have a child than the other. The other partner, often the man, will go along with it for his partner's sake, even though he could well imagine a life without children. When a pregnancy is forced in such cases, for example by the woman's increased desire for sex or by her only wanting to have sex during her fertile days, this could lead to the other partner feeling as if he is only being used for procreation. Of course the same scenario with the roles reversed can also occur.

It can also happen that one or both partners feel that the partnership would remain unfulfilled without a child, that having a child is their very reason for being together, and that this alone will bring them ultimate happiness. If such a couple does not get pregnant within a specific time period it may call their entire relationship into question. If it becomes diagnostically clear that one partner has limited fertility, feelings of guilt and decreased self-worth often arise that weigh more heavily the stronger their desire is to have children. Perhaps an unspoken wish to end the relationship arises. Sometimes in such relationships the desire to have a child is caught up in a hope to stabilize or justify an already unstable relationship—a huge burden for an unborn child to bear.

In order to avoid hurting their partner, many people in such situations simply escape into silence. The topic of having children becomes increasingly taboo, with both partners inwardly grappling with an issue they dare not speak aloud to each other. Both attempt to suppress feelings of grief, helplessness, and anger. The fact that these emotions are left to smolder in secret only makes them more dangerous—and by representing an unspoken conflict, they can lead to the body's rejecting pregnancy.

Unresolved psychological trauma from childhood and young adulthood arising from abuse, abortion, or unprocessed feelings can lead to the psyche simply saying no. Your mind may have internalized horror stories of difficult births, miscarriages, and stillbirths to the extent that it protects itself by not allowing pregnancy at all. Or the psyche may suffer from external burdens: your parents constantly pressuring you to give them a grandchild, your friends always asking when it's finally going to happen, or your sister having already given birth to three healthy children.

These possibilities, along with many others, could lead to psychological barriers preventing pregnancy. Along with the practice of yoga, seeking professional counseling may greatly help you to gain more awareness of and eventually overcome such obstacles.

How Yoga Works

Yoga is derived from the word *yuj*, which means unity. It seeks to unite the trinity of body, mind, and soul. Yoga is both a physical and spiritual practice, and one that has been around for approximately five thousand years, but it is not a religion. You do not have to believe in yoga to feel its positive effects. Yoga is a practically oriented science, meaning that when you practice yoga, you will feel its effects sooner or later. With every passing year yoga is becoming more popular all over the world. In the United States it is estimated that fifteen million people practice yoga—and this number continues to increase. In total, 5 percent of the world's population practices yoga even though it spread outside of India only in the last hundred years.

Yoga works with the entire body: the muscles, organs, and joints. It enlarges lung capacity, energizes the hormonal system, and strengthens the nervous system. Yoga also works on the mind by bringing the right and left sides of the brain into balance. The positive effects upon mind and body that are brought about by the regular practice of yoga have been documented by scientists, with more evidence being recognized each year.

Each yoga practice has five aspects: two physical (pose and movement), two mental (focus and inner concentration), and one physical/mental aspect that connects body and mind: the breath.

The practices in this book are predominantly drawn from kundalini yoga, which I have been teaching for over fifteen years, and to which, despite several detours to other types of yoga, I still feel most strongly connected.

Yoga of Consciousness

Kundalini yoga was brought to the West in 1968 by Yogi Bhajan. It is considered a yoga of consciousness for those who may feel stuck in life because it helps people actively face the daily demands made upon them in a cool, calm, and collected manner. The goal of this self-awareness training is a sustained balance between body, mind, and soul through all aspects of yoga: posture, movement, concentration, breath exercises, meditation, and a healthy lifestyle. Through the combination of these elements, the practice of kundalini yoga leads to a heightened sense of perception, a strong body, and a clear mind.

The long-lived tradition of kundalini yoga originated in north India. Once considered secret knowledge, it was passed down directly from teacher to student. It has only been publicly taught since the 1960s. Yogi Bhajan took the view that in the Age of Aquarius everyone should be free to learn the practice. His decision to make the tradition open to everyone was strongly disapproved of by other yoga masters at the time.

Energy flow plays a central role in kundalini yoga. The term *kundalini* refers to a powerful energy source that rests at the base of the spine. When it is activated through the regular practice of yoga it brings the dichotomy of mind and body into balance, causing a general feeling of harmony. Kundalini yoga is characterized by dynamic, flowing movements, tranquil poses, and rhythmic mantra meditations. The increased flow of life energy that results makes you feel more alert and energetic in your daily routine. Kundalini yoga is therefore not dogmatic but results oriented, and full of meditative practices and techniques that can be easily integrated into your daily schedule.

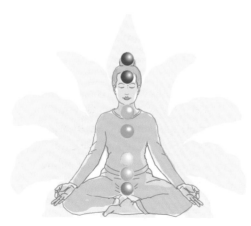

Especially in cases of mental, emotional, and physical stress, kundalini yoga is a particularly effective and fast-acting technique for reaching relaxation and harmonization.

Chakras: Centers of Psycho-Energetic Balance

Chakras are psycho-energetic centers of consciousness, each of them a focal point of energy in the body. Chakras cannot be seen, and as of yet they are not evidenced through scientific imaging techniques. Nonetheless they play a large role in yoga, traditional Chinese medicine, and a number of other alternative medical systems and practices such as acupuncture and acupressure. All of these approaches take as their starting point the idea that humans are primarily energetic beings, and are only secondarily physical beings. It is because we are energetic beings that our body's energy flow has a great influence upon our overall well-being and has the power to initiate all kinds of healing. The essential life energy running through our bodies is called *prana*. Prana is accumulated through our thoughts, nutrition, and breath. Its opposite is *apana,* or *cleansing energy,* which leaves our bodies through exhalation and excretion.

Chakras are traditionally depicted as rotating wheels of energy or as lotus blossoms. When all of one's chakras are cleansed and functioning perfectly, she or he experiences perfect health, happiness, and the ability to live up to her or his full potential.

Chakras are connected through subtle channels of energy called *meridians,* or *nadis.* In this book we take a look at only the seven main chakras, which are positioned along the body's vertical axis (see the figure on the previous page). They lie along the length of *shushumna,* the body's main nadi that runs through the spinal column. Each of the main chakras is associated with a particular color, lotus blossom, sensory function, organ, theme, symbol, aroma, and stone. In addition to the main chakras there are many smaller, secondary chakras that vary greatly and whose numbers can stretch into the thousands.

⋞ Muladhara

The first chakra is called *muladhara,* or the *root chakra,* and it is located at the base of the spine, at the perineum. Its color is red, the element of the earth. Its sensory function is that of smell, and it is symbolized by the four-petalled lotus. It represents stability, security, and fundamental trust. The areas of the body it is connected to are the pelvic organs, large intestine, legs and feet, and all solid parts of the body such as the bones, teeth, and nails. Whoever has an open, unimpeded root chakra usually stands with both feet securely on the ground, is in great health, and feels safe and secure. If one's root chakra is blocked, it often leads to anxiety and depression, stress-related sickness, allergies, or digestive problems.

⋞ Swadhisthana

The second chakra, *swadhisthana,* plays an incredibly important role in fertility. The sexual or sacral chakra lies at the sacrum, the pelvic area between pubis and navel. In Sanskrit, swadhisthana means "place of sweetness." Its color is orange, its element is water, and it is symbolized by the six-petalled lotus. It is associated with the sense of taste, and is connected to sexuality, sensuality, reproduction, creativity, productive life energy, and emotions. The second chakra has an effect upon the pelvic and sacral areas, kidneys (the partner organs), and sexual organs, particularly the ovaries, uterus, gonads, and prostate. It influences all of the bodily fluids, such as blood, lymphatic fluids, tears, and semen. When a person's sexual chakra is functioning well, they live a creative, pleasurable life full of sensuality and satisfaction. They also experience a fulfilled sexual life, and positive, deep connections with members of both sexes. A blocked second chakra leads to an inability to enjoy life, a feeling of weakness, lack of motivation, feelings of jealousy, guilt, and extreme mood swings. It also leads to compulsive sexual behavior, such as sexual addiction or disinterest. It can finally cause physical problems, such as difficulties with menstruation, ovarian and uterine issues, testicular or prostate problems, impotency, venereal disease, or kidney and bladder problems.

To fulfill your wish to have a child, it is especially important to strengthen and cleanse your second chakra.

In addition to practicing yoga exercises, surrounding yourself with aroma essences such as orange and ylang-ylang, getting massages, and enjoying the pleasures of life—from practicing tantra to eating delicious meals, taking walks along the beach, wearing brightly colored clothing, and indulging in fragrant baths—will help you to achieve this.

⪦ Manipura

The third chakra is the *solar plexus chakra,* or *manipura.* Called the "place of gems," it is located about two inches above and behind the navel. Its color is yellow, its element fire, and it is associated with the sense of sight. It is symbolized by the ten-petalled lotus, and it supports personal qualities such as willpower, self-confidence, self-development, and the ability to follow through. It is connected with the digestive system, the stomach, liver, spleen, gallbladder, and the autonomic nervous system. Someone with a strong third chakra works toward accomplishing their goals (and often succeeds) with both energy and enthusiasm, thereby wedding drive with sensitivity. A blocked third chakra can result in low self-esteem, an obsession with power, anger-management problems, eating and/or sleeping issues, hepatitis, or type 2 diabetes.

⋐ Anahata

The fourth chakra is the *heart center, or anahata* (meaning "the untarnished sound"), which is located in the middle of the chest. Its color is pink or light green, its element air, and it is symbolized by a twelve-petalled lotus. It represents unconditional love, openness, tenderness, and healing. It is associated with the heart, lungs, bronchial tubes, skin, arms, hands, and thymus gland. Though it has little to do with physical reproduction, the heart chakra is important for fertility, as it is essential for every couple's relationship and provides the home for a mother's love. It supports sympathy, deep understanding, and the ability to overcome selfish thoughts and actions. A blocked heart chakra leads to relationship problems, bitterness, loneliness,

and, on a physical level, coronary heart disease, circulatory problems, and skin conditions.

⋐ Vishuddha

The fifth chakra is the *throat chakra, or vishuddha,* and it is located in the hollow of the throat. Its color is light blue, its element ether, and it is symbolized by the sixteen-petalled lotus.

It promotes expression, communication, inspiration, and truth. The throat chakra, as the center of truth, is connected to the throat, voice, esophagus, windpipe, neck, jaw, and thyroid. When it is functioning well you will have a high level of verbal competency and expression, be musically talented, and have a beautiful voice with which you are able to sincerely communicate your inner experiences outwardly. A blocked throat chakra can result in inhibition and conformity, stuttering, a hoarse voice, tonsillitis, and thyroid problems.

⋐ Ajna

The sixth chakra is called *ajna,* the *forehead chakra,* or the *third eye,* and it is located between and a little above the eyes. Its color is dark blue, and it is symbolized by the ninety-six petalled lotus. The third eye represents intuition, imagination, awareness, and foresight. It has wide-reaching implications for fertility because it corresponds with the second chakra (just as the first chakra corresponds with the seventh, and the third with the fourth). It is connected to the pituitary gland, the hypothalamus, and the hormonal and nervous systems. Both of these systems play a central role in making one's desire to have children a reality because they control the reproductive organs. Someone with a high-functioning sixth chakra has a good memory, an increased ability to concentrate, mental clarity, an active imagination, and a high level of intuitive awareness. A blocked sixth chakra can cause learning problems, fears, hallucinations, migraine headaches, ear issues, and neurological disorders.

⬙ Sahasrara

The seventh chakra is the *crown chakra*, or *sahasrara*. It represents the "gateway to the universe" and is symbolized by the thousand-petalled lotus. It embodies the universal consciousness, the utmost awareness of existence and spirituality. Its colors are white or violet, and it is connected to the pineal gland, with a protective effect upon the whole body. It is the chakra that, when all other chakras are fully developed and unblocked, can cause enlightenment. It opens the way for the realization that everything is connected, and it brings one's inner and outer worlds into harmonious balance. A blocked crown chakra can lead to feelings of emptiness and lack, to materialistic tendencies, and can cause immune-system deficiencies, multiple sclerosis, and cancer.

"La Luna": The Feminine Moon

Women and their menstrual cycles are strongly connected with the energy of the moon, which, unlike the ever-constant sun, is always changing her appearance: She waxes, becoming rounder, and wanes, in a continuing cycle of change. Sometimes she seems closer, shining as a vast sphere of light clearly in the night sky; then again she becomes small and inconspicuous, a narrow

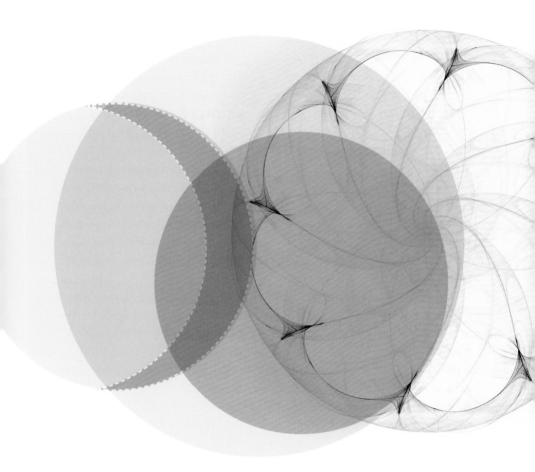

crescent glowing from her far-off home in the heavens.

In yoga it is said that women are beings of the moon and men are beings of the sun. The energy of the sun always remains consistent. Though it is sometimes strong and bright, sometimes hidden behind clouds, sometimes near, sometimes far, unlike the moon it never changes its form.

Women experience extreme hormonal fluctuations, which are often mirrored in the changing of their moods. The effect of the moon, however, goes beyond this. The moon is a symbol for the emotional flow of energy.

The cycle of the moon has an effect upon the earth, upon the tides of the sea, and upon the rhythms of the plant and animal worlds. The energy of the waxing and waning moon affects emotional balance. It is has been determined that under certain natural conditions a woman's menstrual cycle will align itself with the cycle of the moon.

Becoming aware of the moon's effect upon us can bring a sense of relief and empowerment: we are no longer the victims of our own unpredictable emotions or moods, but instead have the power to observe the effect of the moon upon us, and thereby attain greater harmony with ourselves. Women are generally more emotional than men, but also more mutable. Their feelings often change from day to day, even from hour to hour. Yoga and meditation can help you deal with and balance your variety of moods.

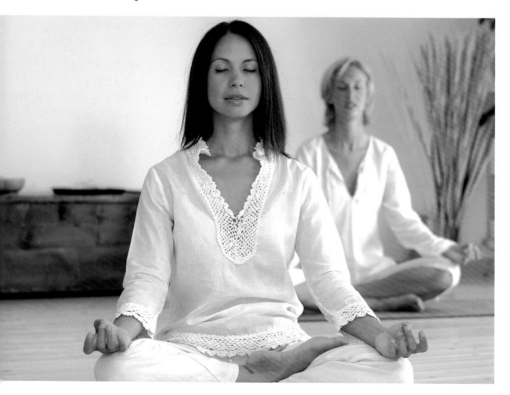

How Yoga Affects Fertility

Ongoing stress wreaks havoc on a woman's hormonal balance, and on a man's sperm count. Yoga, breath, meditation, and relaxation have a healing and balancing effect on the body. Unlike Western medicine yoga does not focus on disease but rather on promoting holistic health, and thereby natural fertility. It is different from normal exercise as well, where movements are often performed in a purely technical way. Yoga integrates body, mind, and soul, encouraging the practice of dedication and mindfulness, which will benefit your body as a future life-giver. Yoga has an especially strong effect on an energetic level; it strengthens and clears the chakras, stimulates the flow of energy in the body, and brings the hormonal and nervous systems into harmony with one another—all of which help to condition the body for pregnancy.

Through the regular practice of yoga, women can increase their chances of becoming pregnant and delivering a healthy baby. The exercises outlined in *Fertility Yoga* stimulate blood circulation in the reproductive organs through light physical training, thereby promoting regular menstruation and ovulation. Men can also increase their fertility through the regular practice of these exercises, as well as through following the other advice to be found here. The fertility of a couple, as the sum of two individuals, can increase substantially when both partners practice yoga and together seek further physical and spiritual development.

Please try to imagine conception as a creative act that can be "egged on" or nudged along by the practice of fertility yoga. It can't guarantee success right away, just as having children can't be planned perfectly in advance. Fertility yoga is a path, in accordance with the following words of wisdom: "There is no way to happiness; happiness is the way." What really helps are patience and tranquility, giving yourself over to the flow of life, and trusting that everything will work out in the end.

CHAPTER 2

PREPARING
FOR PREGNANCY

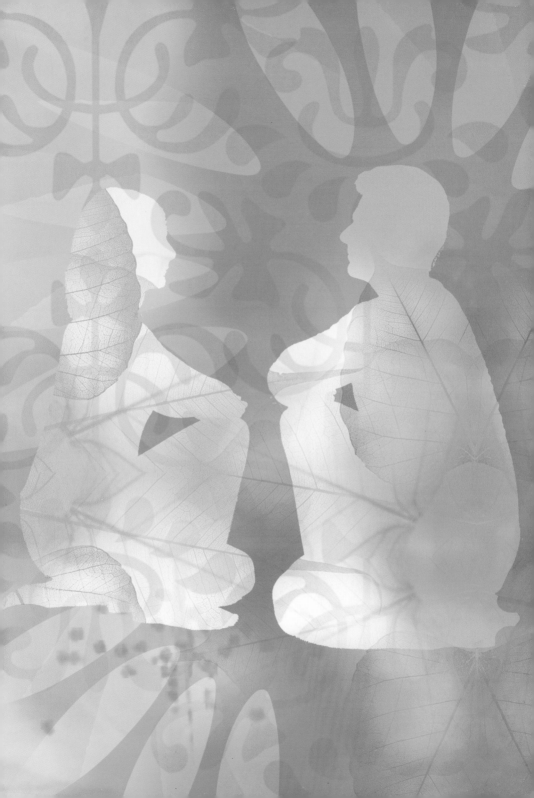

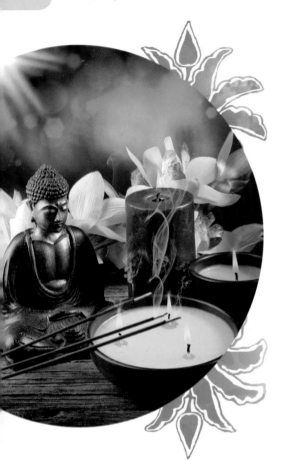

Creating the Optimal Conditions for Body and Mind

Planning a child in advance offers women the opportunity to prepare themselves both physically and mentally in the best way possible. In yoga it is said that the body is the temple of the soul, and as such it should be cleaned, cared for, and kept in order. When a woman becomes pregnant, she is providing her baby a home for nine months—reason enough to prepare that home a bit in advance of the child's arrival. The following recommendations are primarily meant for women but are also relevant for men. Men should pay particular attention to the section "Only for Men: Improving Your Sperm Quality" on page 48.

⊱ Sharpen Your Awareness

It is estimated that around 70 percent of all pregnancies are planned. Even when a woman gets pregnant deliberately, however, she can still experience feelings of ambivalence that fall somewhere between her rational mind and gut feelings. The regular practice of yoga will help you become independent of the conditions of your external reality by helping you find inner strength and certainty. Yoga teaches that a woman should develop a deeper awareness of her body and its functions before becoming pregnant. When this awareness has been developed and the woman is ready to welcome another soul into her body, that is when conception occurs. Her relationship with her partner, with a view toward the future, should be strong and loving. The more understanding the two partners have for each other and their differences, the more secure and protected they will feel in their relationship. Maintaining a supportive, heartfelt connection with your partner in the everyday, through shared interests, conscious connection, and open communication, will prepare the way for conception. The act of making love shouldn't become a routine meant merely for procreation but should represent the height of shared sensual and sexual feelings between you and your partner. Learn to listen to your body more. Learn to trust it more. Even if you don't have a regular menstrual cycle or are unable to measure your ovulation through temperature variation, you can still get pregnant. On the other hand, a picture-perfect menstrual cycle is no guarantee of pregnancy.

⋐ Bring Your Heart, Mind, and Core into Harmony

As was described in the preceding chapter, a person's body, thoughts, and feelings are closely intertwined with one another. The body follows its senses, which are influenced by

its thoughts, and then turns around and expresses its emotions physically. Fear and a need for control are evident in the body, and so is being relaxed and open. Your body mirrors its feelings. The optimal conditions for conception are created when your heart, mind, and core are in unison, and your thoughts, feelings, and actions harmonize with one another. But how can that be achieved with all of the mental and emotional tension that have built up in most people's bodies over the years? Yoga works on a mental as well as a physical level: When you learn to ease your mind and relax your body, emotional release happens automatically. And when you learn to perceive tension in your body through a heightened awareness, the gentle exercises practiced to release that tension have an effect upon your mind and psyche. As soon as you begin trying to have a child, you should start a regular yoga practice, if you haven't done so already.

⋐ Obtain Medical Checkups and Eliminate Unnecessary Medications

Get a thorough checkup from a doctor whom you trust, either to determine that everything is working properly or to learn about how to avoid risks such as high cholesterol, high blood pressure, and diabetes. Pay special attention to all of the "harmless" medications you take and try to avoid them altogether, beginning with aspirin or Tylenol. Antihistamines also have a negative impact on one's fertility as they prevent the implantation of fertilized eggs. Decongestants can dry out the cervical mucus so that it's inhospitable to sperm. Search for alternatives that don't negatively impact fertility. If you have a chronic illness, certain medications are of course vital and can't be replaced; for example, in the case of diabetes, thyroid problems, asthma, or epilepsy. Even undiscovered hyper- or hypothyroidism can negatively affect one's fertility. Consult with your gynecologist or medical specialist, as well as with naturopathic, alternative, or homeopathic doctors, for advice about your individual situation.

Over-the-counter and prescription medications can also negatively affect male fertility. In many cases antidepressants decrease libido, inhibit the ability to achieve erection or ejaculation, and lower sperm quality. Blood pressure medications can decrease the ability of sperm to fertilize an egg. The practice of yoga and its breath exercises have been proven to help combat high blood pressure. Certain medications, such as those for Crohn's disease, inflammatory bowel disease, rheumatism, and arthritis, can also decrease sperm count. Even some natural herbal supplements such as echinacea and gingko have been suspected of decreasing male fertility.

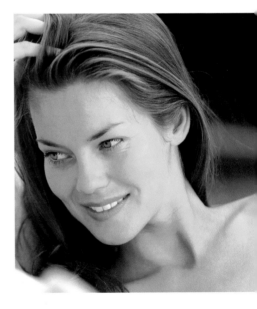

ᔛ Tend to Dental Health

In the old days, women were warned that every child would cost them a tooth. Now we know that undetected problems with a person's teeth or mouth can indeed be the cause of several physical issues. The state of your teeth can actually influence your fertility. Visit a dentist to get your teeth and gums thoroughly examined and cleaned. Gum disease has been suspected of causing premature births and/or low birth weight. If you need further dental work, it is better to have it done before getting pregnant. Continue to implement your own careful teeth-cleaning routine at home to maintain your dental health.

◄ Give Up Smoking and Alcohol

While trying to get pregnant, set aside unhealthy habits like smoking and regular alcohol consumption; that is, try to behave as if you were already pregnant. Smoking leads to the premature aging of a woman's ovaries, brings on menopause an average of two years earlier, and decreases the body's production of estrogen. Smokers also experience a higher risk of miscarriage and premature birth, and often give birth to babies who are underweight. Alcohol and nicotine decrease blood circulation to the ovaries and testicles and adversely affect the metabolism in sex cells. Even if it's going to be

some time before you expect to have children, you should start working to achieve your ideal physical condition now.

◄ Avoid Exposure to Heavy Metals

Exposure to heavy metals represents a particularly strong threat to one's health. Especially if you're trying to get pregnant, you should be careful to avoid contact with heavy metals like lead and mercury, for example at the workplace. These substances have been linked to increased rates of miscarriage, impotence, lower female fertility, and decreased male libido. Before getting pregnant, any heavy metals already existing in the body should be flushed out, which can be a lengthy process. When the body is getting a sufficient supply of vitamins and minerals, it is able to flush a limited quantity of heavy metals out of itself. To facilitate this natural process make sure you are eating enough essential amino acids (found in broccoli, brussels sprouts, spinach, and peas), high-protein foods (like legumes combined with whole grains), as well as enough vitamin B-6 (found in legumes and sunflower seeds, it stimulates the body's ability to heal itself). In addition, several expulsion therapies are available—for example, using algae like chlorella and spirulina—that are better taken under professional supervision.

⮾ Aim for the Right Body Weight

Body weight plays an important role in conception. Being either seriously underweight or overweight is estimated to be responsible for 10 to 25 percent of infertility cases. Having a body weight that is too low can negatively impact the balance of hormones—and no wonder, since about 30 percent of a woman's estrogen, the most important of her sexual hormones, comes from her fat cells. According to a study done at Harvard, underweight women can take up to four times as long to get pregnant as women with a healthy weight. Similarly, being overweight can negatively affect fertility. Having too high a percentage of body fat can throw off a woman's hormonal balance, compromising her ovulation. It can also lead to polycystic ovary syndrome, one of the most common hormonal disorders in women of reproductive age, which is associated with increased levels of androgenic hormones (e.g., testos-

terone), problems with menstruation, and infertility.

Both extremes, having too much or too little body fat, interfere with the body's hormonal balance and decrease fertility. A deviation of only 10 to 15 percent above or below normal body weight can reduce one's chances of having a baby. The ideal percentage of body fat for female fertility is 29 percent. A woman of average height and build should have a body mass index (BMI) between 18.5 and 25 percent. Your BMI can be calculated by taking your body weight in pounds, dividing it by your height in inches squared, and multiplying the result by 703:

$$BMI = \frac{Body\ weight\ (lbs)}{height\ (in^2)} \times 703$$

If you need to gain or lose weight in preparation for pregnancy, it is best to do so using yoga's system of healthy nutrition (see page 33).

It is most difficult for women with eating disorders such as bulimia, binge eating, or anorexia to get pregnant. Anorexic women often have an extremely low BMI that affects their hormone production so significantly that they stop ovulating. Women with bulimia often have a normal body weight, but they suffer from a nutrition deficiency that reduces their fertility and can lead to a hormonal-system imbalance. This also applies to binge eating, which alternates between periods of binging and starving. If you suffer from an eating disorder you should notify your doctor and begin therapy immediately in order to bring your weight and nutrition back into balance—as well as to harmonize your body and mind before attempting to get pregnant.

❦ Resolve Psychological Issues

The brain is actually the "boss" of fertility. It regulates hormone production and controls the reproductive organs. Psychological problems that lead to emotional instability, such as neurosis, psychosis, depression, or personality disorders, can affect your fertility. In addition to the stabilizing effects of yoga, it is recommended that further support be sought for these disorders from a psychotherapist, psychologist, self-help group, or creative therapy. If you already feel unstable, the unnerving process of trying to get pregnant, not to mention pregnancy and caring for a newborn baby, will further overwhelm you.

There are many options for strengthening your psyche that will give you a more-solid foundation for pregnancy and parenthood; you only need to seek them out. Leaving your judgments behind, try a few therapies from the wide variety available, including psychotherapy, cognitive behavioral therapy, family counseling, or emotional-release therapy, and continue with whichever helps you. Courses in nonviolent communication can also be very helpful in improving both your romantic relationship and your relationship with yourself and your environment.

❦ Improve Physical Fitness

Your level of physical fitness plays an important role in your fertility. There are so many ways of being active that even those who hated P.E. classes in school can find something they enjoy doing. Every type of movement can help to prevent the so-called diseases of affluence that afflict our modern-day society. Moderate but regular exercise burns excess fat, supports fertility, strengthens the cardiovascular system, and increases energy levels. It also helps you cope with the emotional challenges involved in

trying to have a child because it strengthens the psyche.

Too much exercise, however, negatively influences a woman's fertility because it can cause an acute stress response. Excessive physical training can lead to fallopian tube dysfunction. While attempting to get pregnant it is best to exercise moderately through activities such as swimming, water gymnastics, walking, light weight training, stretching, Pilates, and of course yoga. These types of exercises optimally prepare the body for pregnancy and birth by strengthening the abdominal, pelvic, and back muscles. It is recommended that a person undertake such exercises thirty minutes daily, four to five days per week.

As an added bonus, exercising regularly for at least one year before getting pregnant reduces a woman's risk of developing gestational diabetes by 50 percent. If you stay moderately active during pregnancy the risk decreases even further. Finally, pregnancy constitutes an enormous drain on a woman's body, which is best counteracted by being in good physical condition.

Strengthen Your Immune System

Signs of a compromised immune system are frequent infections, chronic fatigue, or chronic allergies. Colds that never seem to go away are a signals that the body is trying to detoxify itself. Every infection is a misguided attempt by the body to eliminate toxins. You can support your body's defense system with good nutrition, regular exercise in the fresh air, trips to the sauna, healing fasts, herbal medicine, and specific yoga practices. (If you speak German, you can find tips for the latter in my book *Nie mehr Schnupfen & Co: Yoga für das Immunsystem* [No More Sniffles: Yoga for the Immune System].) You can get professional help to permanently increase your immune defenses through homeopathy, which determines the person's basic constitutional type and suggests compatible treatments after a careful evaluation of her medical history.

Improve Your Living Environment

It is important to establish good conditions in your home environment, because that is where you probably spend the most time. To eliminate potentially harmful chemicals switch to using "green" or earth-friendly cleaning products and natural cosmetics. Examine your house or apartment for questionable materials that could harm you and your unborn child. From an energetic standpoint, consider hiring a building biologist to test your home for electromagnetic radiation, underground water veins, and e-rays (earth rays). Simple measures such as changing the position of your bed, using cork mats to deflect e-rays, or installing a switch against electromagnetic radiation can improve the home environment.

Find Balance

Find a balance between the opposite poles of yin and yang. Yin represents the feminine principle and yang the masculine. They are conceptualized in yoga as *Shakti,* the soft, warm pole at the perineal base of the spine, and *Shiva,* the hard, cool pole at the top of the head. It is between these two opposites that our entire life is played out. The contrasting conditions of relaxation and tension depend on each other and should be kept in balance.

Avoid the extremes of being constantly overburdened or lying around all day doing nothing. Seek a harmonious exchange between work and free time, waking and sleeping, tension and relaxation, stillness and movement, play and seriousness, nearness and distance, enjoyment and discipline, and warmth and cold. Nearly all human experience falls into these categories, and we naturally aim for balance. Finding your own personal balance is a prerequisite for living a happy, healthy, and fulfilled life.

Enhancing Fertility Through Nutrition

"You are what you eat" is a well-known proverb. Nutrition has an enormous influence on our health and well-being. The pharmaceutical industry would probably go bankrupt if the entire world ate well, because proper nutrition can prevent and heal disease. For many people it seems easier to eat in an irregular and unhealthy way, and to simply take pills later on to combat the resulting ailments and disease.

Even women who have never taken an interest in nutrition will often become more sensitive to the issue once they start thinking about getting pregnant. They want to give their unborn child the best possible start in life. Proper nutrition can promote your natural fertility—and certain foods and a few significant dietary supplements can even help you to get pregnant sooner. Nutrition and fertility are intimately related. If a woman's body is not given the proper nutrition, it goes into emergency mode, and the first thing it shuts off is its reproductive system so as to avoid being overburdened with a pregnancy.

Whenever possible, eat fresh, natural foods, and choose, prepare, and consume them mindfully. Ideally, eat a balanced diet with plenty of variety. Give preference to fruits and vegetables produced locally, and to whole-grain products as opposed to highly refined grains. Whenever possible choose organic foods. Eat fish regularly, and little or no meat. Avoid industrially produced products, sweets, and stimulants such as caffeine. Nourish yourself through the yogic principle: Don't live to eat, but eat to live. Yet don't entirely deprive yourself of what you enjoy. Eating is supposed to be fun—it's a sensual pleasure, just like sex. Don't give up your favorite foods entirely, either in the literal or figurative sense. Carefully and consciously choose your vices, instead of swearing off everything you enjoy.

What follows are a few dietary principles for enhancing fertility.

⬱ Whole Grains for Ovulation

Yogic nutrition has always espoused a well-balanced, vegetarian diet with a lot of vegetables, fruits, mung beans, sprouts, and whole grains. Eating complex carbohydrates such as whole-grain products, fruits, and vegetables can improve ovulation, while products with white flour can hinder it because they increase blood sugar levels and upset hormonal balance. Try several whole-grain products like oats, whole-grain wheat, amaranth, spelt, cornmeal, brown rice, millet, buckwheat, and pearl barley.

In terms of fertility, millet is a wonder grain. It's gluten free, so it's good for those with allergies and sensitivities, and it helps to balance blood sugar and insulin levels. It exerts an overall positive influence on hormonal balance. People with thyroid issues should be careful using millet as it can cause excessive production of thyroid hormone.

⋚ The "Three-Thirds" Rule

If you're a pure vegetarian, you should read a book about yogic nutrition that recommends special recipes with increased protein levels for before and during your pregnancy. See the Resources section for recommended books.

For nonvegetarians, here is an easy rule, especially for women who are overweight: Make sure to get about one-third of your total calories from protein (especially from poultry, fish, and yogurt); one-third from complex carbohydrates like whole-grain products, legumes, and green vegetables; and one-third from unsaturated fatty acids, like those found in nuts, olive oil, and avocados.

⋚ No Low-Fat Dairy Products

Nutritional experts usually advise eating low-fat dairy products. While trying to get pregnant, however, it is advisable to eat dairy products daily with a minimum fat content of 3.5 percent. According to an American study of eighteen thousand women, the consumption of two servings of dairy products daily—for example, a glass of whole milk and a serving of full-fat yogurt—reduced the women's chances of infertility by 50 percent. Researchers suspect that the hormones estrogen and progesterone contained in the milk

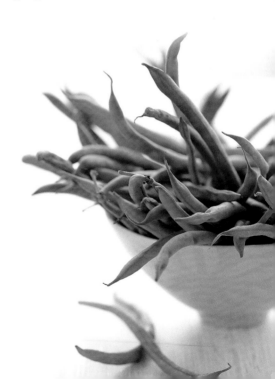

actually accumulate on a woman's fat molecules, enhancing fertility. Eating reduced-fat dairy products means you reduce your intake of these important hormones, while the levels of other hormones, such as androgens, insulin-mimicking growth factors, and prolactin, none of which support fertility, remain the same. An interesting fact: Vegans have an 80 percent less chance of having twins than vegetarians, possibly because the latter eat milk products.

Plant Sources of Iron

Women trying to get pregnant should pay close attention to their iron levels, as a lack of iron in the worst-case scenario can lead to infertility. Even though red meat contains a lot of iron, women who want to get pregnant should increase their intake of plant sources of iron. According to a study done at Harvard, too much iron intake from animal sources can actually hinder pregnancy. Women with a high intake of iron from plant sources, on the other hand, can improve their fertility. Good plant sources of iron include sesame, dried apricots, wheat bran, oats, flaxseed, amaranth, spinach, broccoli, lentils, millet, green beans, and peas. Vitamin C improves iron absorption. Try sprinkling lemon juice over your meal, and avoid drinking any accompanying black or green tea, which can diminish iron absorption.

Alternatively, you can take iron supplements and multivitamin tablets to improve your chances of getting pregnant.

Vegetable Sources of Protein

Getting enough protein is important, but most people get too much of it, especially if they eat meat. When your protein need is fulfilled primarily through vegetable sources like beans, nuts, and peas, you increase your chances of getting pregnant. According to a study done at Harvard, the chances of infertility can increase by eating red meat once a day. Soy is a good source of protein, but it is better to avoid eating soy products during your fertile days (for more on this topic see below).

Vitamin E for Ovaries or Testes

Vitamin E plays an important role in reproduction: It helps the fertilized egg implant in the womb and thereby sustains pregnancy, and it increases the mobility and life span of sperm. Vitamin E is found in wheat germ, green leafy vegetables, peas, beans, sesame, sunflower seeds, wheat germ oil, and all whole grains.

It can also be taken through nutritional supplements, and is recommended to help prepare both men and women for fertilization.

⋐ Folic Acid for Hormones

Folic acid is a B vitamin that helps a woman's fertilized egg successfully implant in her uterus. In addition, it is necessary for the body's production of the female reproductive hormones estrogen and progesterone, as well as follicle-stimulating hormone (FSH). It therefore makes sense to start taking folic acid as soon as you decide to try for pregnancy. Folic acid can also reduce the chances of abnormal development during the first trimester of pregnancy. The baby needs folic acid to form vital parts of its developing body, including its brain, bones, organs, and skin.

Folic acid can be found in green vegetables like lettuce, spinach, broccoli, cabbage, beans, and peas, as well as in oranges and grapes. Pregnant women need 50 percent more folic acid (600 micrograms) than women who aren't pregnant (400 micrograms). Folic acid can also be taken as a nutritional supplement.

⋐ Zinc for Ovulation

Zinc is a dietary mineral that, in addition to folic acid and iron, plays an important role in reproduction and regular ovulation. It is contained in most multivitamins, but you should pay attention to the amount: Aim for 8 to 11 milligrams during pregnancy.

⋐ Vitamin B-12 for Vegans and Vegetarians

A B-12 deficiency can lead to infertility, impede ovulation, and reduce the ability of a fertilized egg to implant in the uterus. Since eggs and meat are the main sources of vitamin B-12, vegans and strict vegetarians should take dietary supplements.

⋐ No Soy in the Middle of Your Menstrual Cycle

Yogic nutrition normally recommends eating a lot of soy products. Soy contains isoflavonoids, biologically active compounds that are identified as phytohormones, or plant hormones. Phytohormones have an effect on a woman's body that is similar to (but weaker than) her own estrogen. For women going through menopause, phyto-hormones have a positive effect in helping to balance the body's decrease in hormone production. This harmonizing effect can begin long before actual menopause. Women who are trying to get pregnant, however, should be careful with soy products, especially avoiding them around the time of ovulation. The reason: One of the phytoestrogens, genistein, has recently been suspected of sabotaging sperm as they swim toward the egg.

⋐ Good Fats, Bad Fats, Trans Fats

Consuming unsaturated fatty acids increases a woman's chances of pregnancy by decreasing inflammation and reducing insulin sensitivity, two factors important to hormone balance. Monounsaturated fatty acids are found in olives, peanuts, and canola oil, as well as in avocados, cashews, almonds, sesame seeds, and pumpkin seeds. Polyunsaturated fatty acids, which contain omega-3 fatty acids, are found in fish that have a fat content greater than 10 percent, such as sardines, eel, herring, tuna, salmon,

mackerel, and cod. Plant sources of omega-3 fatty acids include flaxseed, walnuts, sunflower oil, thistle oil, and corn oil. The consumption of foods containing these kinds of fats supports the health of both the heart and the greater circulatory system. At the same time, remember that some fish, such as mackerel (king), marlin, orange roughy, shark, swordfish, tilefish, and tuna (bigeye, ahi), contain high levels of mercury or other harmful substances, such as polychlorinated biphenyls (PCBs), which can accumulate in the body. You should start avoiding fish that can contain high levels of such substances a year before your planned pregnancy.

You should also sharply reduce your intake of trans fats. Trans fats are mostly found in packaged (processed) foods, fried products, and baked goods that use partially hydrogenated oils, such as French fries, potato chips, and various kinds of shortening, frying grease, and margarine. This harmful fat is also found in many commercially prepared cookies, cakes, and chocolate. On a package's ingredients, trans fats will usually be listed as "partially hydrogenated fat or oil." Although the human body is able to metabolize trans fats, an intake higher than about 3.4 grams per day increases the levels of "bad" cholesterol (LDL cholesterol) and triglycerides in the blood, especially for women. Triglycerides are primarily made from saturated fats, and blood levels that are too high increase a person's risk for heart disease, arteriosclerosis, and strokes, and decreases fertility. A study at Harvard determined that a daily intake of only 4 grams of trans fats substantially decreases fertility. The amount of trans fats contained in one serving of French fries from a fast food restaurant is more than double this number.

Caffeine, Sugar, and Cinnamon

The best beverage for people trying to conceive is the same as it is for everyone else: pure water. Drink at least two liters of water a day to ensure the proper functioning of internal organs and to efficiently expel toxins and metabolic waste. If you can't or won't completely give up drinking coffee or tea, at least decrease your intake of them, and start thinking of them as stimulants. Caffeine stresses the body, makes you jittery, and interferes with your normal sleep pattern—all of which have a negative effect on fertility. Studies have shown that the body can tolerate a moderate amount of caffeine, but more than 300 milligrams daily, equivalent to the amount contained in about three cups of coffee, decreases fertility and increases risk of miscarriage. All beverages containing caffeine should therefore be avoided. The high amount of sugar in many such beverages also has a negative effect on blood sugar and insulin levels, and therefore on hormone levels. Yogis advise drinking noncarbonated water (because carbonation is acidic) and yogi tea. Most stores now carry a wide assortment of yogi teas, and you can drink any of them without worry. Yogi tea cleanses the liver and stimulates the hormonal and nervous systems. The classical yogi tea also contains a bit of cinnamon. Recent studies have found that cinnamon increases cells' sensitivity to insulin, prevents a rapid increase in blood sugar levels after eating, and helps to balance hormone levels.

⋐ The Yogic Green Diet for Promoting Fertility

In the months before getting pregnant, future parents should cleanse their bodies with at least one seven-day yogic green diet. This diet is deacidifying, cleanses the liver and other organs, clears toxins from the body, and remedies skin problems. It can be undertaken for up to forty days but should be stopped before becoming pregnant as detoxification should be avoided during pregnancy.

It is called the green diet because only green foods are allowed, ideally organic ones. Acceptable foods include all varieties of lettuce, steamed leafy green vegetables, avocados, broccoli, zucchini, cucumbers, green bell peppers, kohlrabi, green beans, peas, artichokes, celery, cabbage, Brussels sprouts, Chinese cabbage—whatever is available. You can eat these vegetables raw or steamed and garnished with fresh herbs or olive oil. You can also include green fruits such as honeydew melon, green apples, green grapes, pears, kiwis, olives, and mung beans. In case you're yearning for protein, you may eat a handful of nuts per week or a portion of grains, but no more. Drink as much yogi tea, water, and vegetable broth as you wish. At the end of your fast, you should begin with eating fruit, then reintroduce grains, and dairy products last of all.

Natural Remedies That Promote Fertility

When trying to get pregnant, it's a good idea to pay attention to nature's pharmacy. It offers diverse means of promoting and supporting fertility naturally—especially in women. This section describes several fertility-promoting herbal remedies.

⋐ Monk's Pepper (*Agnus Castus*)

Monk's pepper, also called chaste tree, is indigenous to the humid areas of Asia and the Mediterranean region. The tall shrubs have fragrant blossoms that grow into fruit. When dried, it is used medicinally. Monk's pepper has been known for quite a while for its ability to decrease premenstrual cramps and to alleviate heavy menstrual bleeding and cramps. It can also harmonize irregular menstrual cycles. It is less known for its proven ability to increase one's chances of pregnancy. Monk's pepper regulates the hormone levels and thereby supports regular ovulation. It also promotes the successful uterine implantation of the fertilized egg. The plant's effectiveness has been proven in clinical trials. In one study at the University of Heidelberg, in Germany, women who took monk's pepper were twice as likely to get pregnant as women who took placebo. The plant's active agents influence the release of the neurotransmitter dopamine, thereby normalizing the milk-producing hormone prolactin in the pituitary gland. Women with PMS often have increased prolactin levels, a hormone that is more widely distributed in the body during pregnancy and lactation. An increased level of prolactin can, however, lead to the cessation of ovulation. As with all other medicinal plants, it takes from several weeks to six months for Monk's pepper to deliver its full effect.

False Unicorn (*Chaemlirium Luterum*)

This healing plant is indigenous to North America, east of the Mississippi, and was used by the Native Americans to deal with gynecological issues. The herb regulates a woman's menstrual cycle and stimulates egg maturation. It is also effective in combating impotency in men. It is thought to support the development of ovarian follicles and to heal infertility that stems from ovarian problems.

Chinese Angelica (*Angelica Sinensis*)

Chinese angelica regulates hormonal balance. In Asia it is used as a medicinal herb for gynecological problems and for regulating disruptions of the menstrual cycle. The herb achieves this effect by increasing circulation to the uterus.

⪜ Ginger
(Zingiberis Rhizoma)

Ginger stimulates circulation, reduces inflammation, and relieves cramps. It helps with delayed menstrual bleeding, relieves pain experienced during ovulation, and strengthens the reproductive organs. Ginger is highly valued by yogis because it strengthens the immune and nervous systems.

GINGER WITH LEMON

Peel and cut into small pieces a one-inch piece of ginger root. In a small, clean pot, heat about four cups of water; add the ginger, and let it simmer on low heat for half an hour. Squeeze the juice from half a lemon into the mix, and drink the resulting ginger-lemon water throughout the day.

⪜ Lady's Mantle
(Alchemilla Vulgaris)

This plant is found all over Europe, in eastern North America, in Greenland, and in Asia from the Caucasus and Himalayas to Siberia. Its name comes from the shape of its leaves, which look like a lady's coat from bygone days. Lady's mantle balances the hormonal system, regulates the menstrual cycle, and treats menstrual discomfort. Also known as the woman's herb, it improves circulation to the pelvic organs. Lady's mantle is especially helpful with menstrual-cycle issues related to being overweight. It promotes egg maturation and helps to build the lining of the uterus.

⪜ Raspberry Leaves
(Rubi Idaei Folium)

Raspberry leaves help to regulate hormones in cases of menstrual problems. They also strengthen the uterine and pelvic muscles. The leaves are usually made into a tea that relaxes the uterus, and is therefore often recommended for menstrual cramps. The relaxing of the uterine muscles improves circulation, aiding in the formation of the uterine lining.

⪜ Fertility Teas

Several varieties of tea both promote fertility and support the cleansing and strengthening processes that are triggered by the yoga exercises described in this book. Yoga warms and energizes the pelvic organs; tea maintains and sustains that warmth. Here are recipes for three different teas.

TWO-PHASE FERTILITY TEA

During the first half of your menstrual cycle:

2 parts raspberry leaves (contains estrogen-mimicking elements)

1 part mugwort (promotes ovulation and detoxification)

1 part elderflower (supports follicle-stimulating hormone, FSH)

1 part sage (estrogen-mimicking effect)

During the second half of your menstrual cycle:

2 parts lady's mantle (regulates the corpus luteum)

1 part yarrow (progesterone-mimicking effect)

1 part stinging nettle (supports the evacuation of impurities, contains iron)

Add one tablespoon of tea to one cup of boiling water and let it seep for fifteen minutes. Drink four to five cups per day.

HARMONY TEA FOR WOMEN

This tea strengthens and heals the female reproductive organs and harmonizes sexual function.

Mix raspberry, strawberry, and blackberry leaves, yarrow, and lady's mantle in equal parts.

Add one tablespoon of the blend to three cups of boiling water, and let the tea steep for ten minutes. Drink it throughout the day.

POWER TEA FOR MEN

Tea made from a mix of equal parts oregano, thyme, wild thyme, goldenrod, and mullein has a positive effect for men. It strengthens the masculine reproductive organs and stimulates metabolism and hormonal balance.

Add one tablespoon of the mix to three cups of water, bring it to a boil, and let it steep for ten minutes.

Additional Alternative Therapies for Fertility

Alternative medicine, also called complementary medicine, offers many ways of gently enhancing fertility and supporting the body before and during pregnancy.

☙ Homeopathic Support

The aim of homeopathy is to strengthen one's life energy and improve the body's functioning and natural fertility. Seek out a classical homeopathic physician who will spend at least an hour with you. She or he will review your medical history to determine your basic constitutional type and from there will develop a remedy tailored to your needs.

Certain homeopathic remedies are often used for promoting a woman's fertility, including monk's pepper (*Agnus castus*) and lady's mantle (*Alchemilla vulgaris*), mentioned above, as well as pulsatilla, sepia (squid), and ovaria comp, which stimulates both hormone production and sexual desire. Ovaria comp, a mixture of several healing herbs, affects egg maturation. If ovulation hasn't occurred by the fourteenth day of your cycle this remedy can help to trigger earlier ovulation. It also improves the quality and quantity of cervical mucus. Ovaria comp is taken in the first half of the menstrual cycle, until ovulation. It should be avoided if you are already taking conventional ovulation-promoting medications.

The homeopathic remedy bryophyllum can help in cases when the second half of the menstrual cycle is

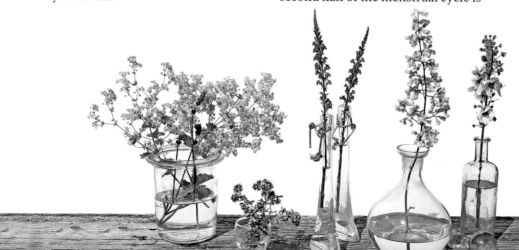

too short. It is only taken in the days following ovulation. Bryophyllum has an effect similar to progesterone, improving the construction of the uterine lining and supporting the fertilized egg's implantation in the uterus.

If you seek to get pregnant using homeopathic means, have patience—as is the case with all the methods suggested in this book. To find the remedy that works best for the individual, a homeopathic physician must conduct an extensive analysis of the patient's or couple's situation. The first homeopathic remedy tried often doesn't work right away; sometimes problems are even exacerbated at the beginning. In homeopathy, when a condition gets worse before it gets better it is considered a sign that the remedy is the correct one.

Traditional Chinese Medicine

Traditional Chinese medicine (TCM), by considering people holistically, aims to bring body and mind into harmonious balance. The process of diagnosis includes studying the tongue and the pulse; treatment includes making nutritional recommendations and using healing herbs. Herbs prescribed for fertility issues might include ginseng, which balances the menstrual cycle, and sage palmetto, which can help with polycystic ovary syndrome, a condition affecting an estimated five to seven million women in the United States.

TCM also helps men bring their bodies into balance, improving fertility.

Increasing Fertility with Acupuncture

Like yoga, acupuncture is based on energetic principles. Both systems help to clear blockages in the meridians, or nadis—the body's energy superhighways—thereby increasing health, well-being, and fertility. A course of acupuncture usually lasts three months; the physician treats the patient with ultra-fine needles one to two times per week, followed by a break to see how the patient's body reacts. According to some studies, acupuncture improves a woman's fertility. It stimulates the nervous system to produce natural sedatives like beta-endorphins and ensures regular ovulation. The increased energy flow promoted by acupuncture also increases circulation to the uterus.

Men also benefit from acupuncture, which increases the number and mobility of sperm. A German study showed that after five weeks of regular acupuncture treatment undertaken by infertile male subjects, the number of structural abnormalities in their sperm decreased significantly and their sperm counts rose. During the three-year study, more than 20 percent of the participants became fathers.

⮂ Acupressure

Acupressure, the practice of stimulating specifically targeted massage points, is closely related to acupuncture. You can easily treat yourself to improve the functioning of your pelvic organs by massaging certain acupressure points. You can use lighter or firmer pressure to influence the level of circulation of both blood and lymphatic fluid to the area. In this way you can enhance the body's drainage and detoxification processes. You don't need any special knowledge of anatomy to practice acupressure, simply an open mind.

1. Stand and place your index and middle fingers on your lower back; locate the tailbone and sacrum, which lie an inch or so above the crease of your buttocks. To the sides you should be able to feel two small indentations. Massage these softly. If you like, you can use a mild massage oil such as almond oil.

2. Sit on the floor and place the soles of your feet comfortably apart, letting your knees fall open. Use your thumbs to feel for the point underneath and behind your ankle bone on the inside of the foot. Stimulating this acupressure point relieves several problems with the genital tract. Massage it using gentle or firmer pressure, as you wish.

3. Still sitting, bring your knees up in front of you so that the soles of your feet are flat on the floor. Place your thumb and forefinger on either side of the back of your heel. Put pressure on the point behind the ankle bone on the

outside of the foot, and massage the area softly or more firmly. Stimulating this point helps to clear up problems in the pelvic region.

4. Remain in a sitting position. With your forefinger or thumb apply pressure to the point located on the outside edge of the nail on the pinky toe. Stimulating this point provides relief for PMS that can be accompanied by gas, tension, and difficult-to-manage feelings.

5. Keeping your feet in front of you, touch the point between your pinky toe and the one next to it with your forefinger, feeling for a small recess. This recess is a massage point that relieves several difficulties in the lower body and genital tract. Massage it softly or more firmly, as you prefer.

Aromatherapy

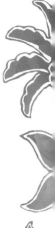
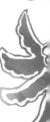

Aromatherapy can have a positive influence on your fertility. Civilizations as far back as ancient Egypt were distilling essential oils from plants and applying them to the body and face for healing purposes during religious ceremonies. Essential oils are pure, fluid herbal essences. They are made from several different parts of the plant. They stimulate the sense of smell, improve one's mood, and have a positive effect on one's overall mental and physical well-being. They can be used as bath additives, massage oils, or room scents. Because essential oils are highly concentrated, you should only use them drop by drop. Never apply them directly to your skin; first mix them with a neutral "base" oil. To stimulate fertility use essential oils such as musk, ginger, vanilla, patchouli, cinnamon, cloves, basil, and geranium, according to your personal preferences.

Only for Men: Improving Your Sperm Quality

To maintain or improve their fertility men should pay close attention to their weight, eating a well-balanced diet containing plenty of vitamins, minerals, and fiber. For a man's testes to produce enough testosterone and an adequate sperm count, his body needs to get enough vitamin C, vitamin E, vitamin B-12, beta-carotene, folic acid, selenium, and zinc. If he isn't getting enough of any of these nutrients he may experience a decrease in sperm quality.

Overweight men suffer from noticeably lower sperm quality. In the past it was assumed that the lifespan of sperm was between seventy and ninety days; newer studies have shown that it is only about forty-two days. That means any measures taken to improve sperm quality actually have a much quicker effect than previously thought. The number of healthy sperm needed for fertilization to occur is presumed to be about twenty million sperm cells per milliliter (cc) of semen. If a man's sperm is less concentrated than this, the probability of fertilization diminishes. Furthermore, it turns out that men have a biological clock: They can theoretically have children at an advanced age, but most recent studies have shown that genetic defects in sperm rapidly increase beginning in the mid-thirties. Another study has shown that increased age of the father is associated with an increased risk of autism, schizophrenia, dwarfism, Down syndrome, and other genetic disorders. After the age of forty, a man's fertility steadily and rapidly decreases. Not only does his sperm count decrease, but the sperm that are present lose mobility, leading to what doctors call "lazy sperm." If possible, men shouldn't wait too long to become fathers.

Here are a few other pointers to enhance your fertility.

⬟ Consider Supplementing L-Carnitine

Decreased sperm count and mobility can often be attributed to a lack of essential nutrients like L-carnitine. L-carnitine is partly synthesized in the body from two essential amino acids, lysine and methionine, but its primary supply comes from food intake. Meat and dairy products are especially high in L-carnitine.

It is also available as a nutritional supplement. As such, it is often used in efforts to lose weight because it burns fat. It is an important component of energy metabolism.

Organs such as the muscles and heart contain L-carnitine. But sperm have the most L-carnitine of any cells in the entire body, containing about two thousand times as much as blood cells. It is thought that the amount of L-carnitine in the epididymis, the tube that connects the testicle with the vas deferens, is directly related to the number, mobility, and maturity of sperm cells.

Vegetarians and men with fertility problems should take micronutrient supplements of L-carnitine. These supplements often also contain L-arginine, which improves sperm quality. L-arginine is a semi-essential amino acid that can improve fertility in two ways: It improves a man's ability to achieve erection and increases the number and mobility of his sperm.

⋐ Maintain the Right Temperature

The production of sperm requires a temperature between 93.9 and 95.9 degrees Fahrenheit—slightly below normal body temperature. That's why the testes are housed outside the body cavity. Men who want to increase their fertility should make sure to keep their testicles cool when they undertake any kind of physical exertion such as working out. Avoid wearing fitness clothes that don't breathe, such as tight pants. After working out, you should wash your testicles in cool water and ideally let them air dry—or at the very least wear loose, breathable cotton clothes. The classical yogis recommend wearing wide, loose underwear called *katcheras*, but comfortable boxer shorts also work well. Avoid saunas, steam rooms, and hot baths while trying to conceive.

Water beds have also played a role in inhibiting men's efforts to conceive, as the heat generated by the warmer water can reduce male fertility. For the same reason you should use sheets made of natural fibers and avoid synthetics.

⋐ Limit Participation in Certain Sports

Certain types of sports, like bicycling, should be avoided or at least limited while trying to get your partner pregnant. Some bicycle seats, especially older ones, are made in such a way that they apply pressure to the nerve-rich perineum, the area between the anus and testicles. From an energetic standpoint the perineum represents the root chakra. If this area is subjected to prolonged pressure several hours per week, it can lead to numbness and circulation problems in the genitalia, and, for some men, to erectile dysfunction. Most of these symptoms are temporary; however, in some cases they can be chronic and irreversible, requiring surgery. If you're a cyclist, make sure your bike saddle doesn't have a "nose" and is constructed so that it doesn't damage your reproductive organs. Bicycling should be restricted to three hours per week for men wanting to conceive.

Contact sports like football, baseball, and handball, as well as combat sports like boxing, karate, and judo, carry a higher risk of injuring the testicles and groin. Blunt force trauma to these areas can damage sperm production. If you don't want to give up these sports altogether, you should at least wear groin-protective gear while you're attempting to conceive, although the increased heat gener-

ated by the gear has the potential to decrease your fertility.

⇐ Avoid Medications for Erectile Dysfunction

Medications that increase erectile potency should be avoided while attempting to have a child. An Irish study determined that even one 100 milligram dose of Viagra can cause sperm to prematurely shed their acrosome cap. The acrosome is composed of a double membrane containing certain enzymes needed to break through the egg cell's protective layer. If it is shed prematurely it is no longer available when needed to fertilize the egg.

⇐ Watch Pornography

An Australian study has shown that watching pornographic photos or films can increase male fertility. Semen samples drawn from men right after looking at pornography demonstrated greater numbers and increased mobility of sperm. This astonishing result is theoretically based on the fact that human males, like other mammals, produce better sperm when placed in situations of (supposed) competition to win over the desired female.

⋐ Get Fresh Air

Poor air quality has a negative effect not only on your lungs but also on your fertility. A study conducted in California showed that increased levels of smog and ozone in the air were directly associated with lower sperm counts. Men living in the countryside therefore have an advantage over men living in cities. It is recommended that you spend the summer months (when ozone levels are higher) concentrating on indoor sports, make trips to the countryside more often, and, if you live in an area with high smog levels, install air filters in your home.

⋐ Get a Checkup

A common cause of male infertility is a *varicocele,* a widening of the veins along the spermatic cord that holds up the testicles. Essentially forming a varicose vein, the widening usually occurs on the left side but sometimes happens on both sides. Approximately 15 percent of men have a varicocele—often without knowing

it. Only after it has existed for long enough to produce pronounced evidence will you begin to notice tension and swelling in the area. Varicose veins in a man's testicles decrease his sperm quality. The resulting reduced circulation and blood stagnation can also overheat the testicle. If you have a varicocele you should have it surgically corrected—at the latest when you start to feel pain. Doing so will usually increase your sperm quality.

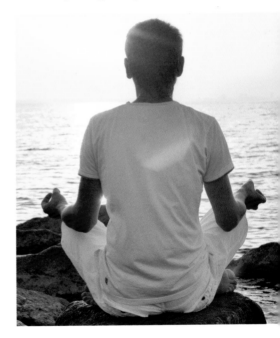

CHAPTER 3

YOGA POSES THAT PROMOTE FERTILITY

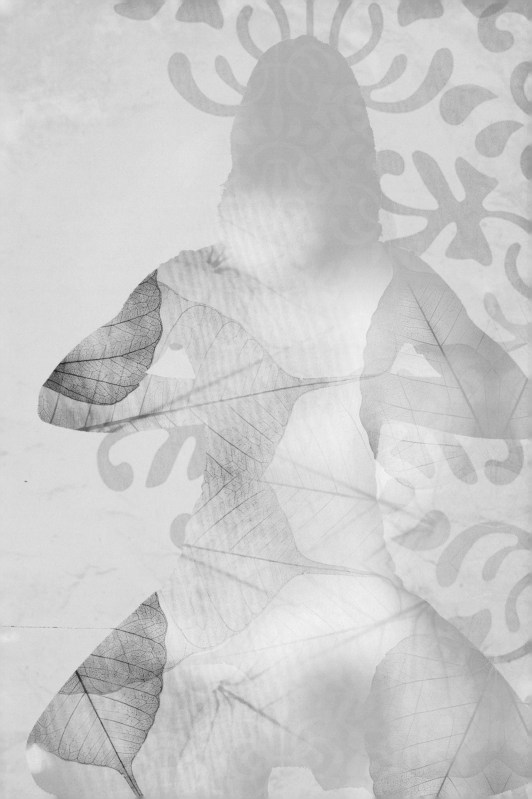

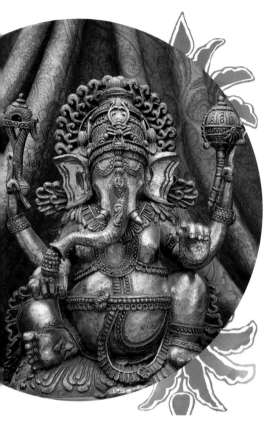

Taking Responsibility for Yourself

Now we come to the heart of the book: Fertility yoga, a practice that stimulates life force and vital energy. Fertility yoga differs greatly from medical fertility treatments, which often rob a couple of their energy and leave them weak, needy, and dependent. By contrast, fertility yoga makes you an active agent in influencing your reproduction. Conceiving a child is a highly creative act.

You should regularly, if possible daily, get onto your yoga mat to get to know your body better, to make it stronger and more flexible, and to facilitate the flow of your life force. You will feel more fit, more relaxed, healthier, and just better overall. If you're actively trying to prepare for pregnancy and stimulate your fertility, adopt the attitude that you're taking increasingly greater responsibility for yourself. There is a difference between putting your reproduction in the hands of experts and taking it into your own hands. When you take responsibility for yourself and your body you become stronger and more clear-minded, and hopefully you will soon be holding your own child in your arms.

I'd like to offer an example from my life. When I was pregnant with my daughter, I had already started practicing a little yoga, had read a book on yoga for pregnant women, and had taken a class on preparing for birth. I visualized bringing my daughter yogically into the world through breath exercises and asanas. Even so, as the pain of labor set in I was surprised by its force. The first contractions unfortunately proved to be just the beginning. As an unrelenting midwife told me, "The real pain hasn't even started." I spent hours in the labor room at the clinic, not allowed to eat or drink, unable to sleep, and becoming increasingly weaker and disheartened. After more than thirty-six hours I was totally exhausted and begged for an epidural, which in 1993 meant completely losing the ability to move. So there I was, with tubes in my hands and a catheter in my spine, attached to the fetal monitor, and being heaved back and forth every twenty minutes so that my baby's head would finally get in position. Surrounded by beeping machines, I lay helpless on my back. As my heartbeat became fainter and fainter over the next ten hours, my daughter was abruptly pulled out with forceps. Looking back, it felt more like a "delivery" than a "birth."

Four and a half years later, with the arrival of my second child, things were different. This time I had already decided to have a cesarean section because my son had remained in a transverse position despite the yoga poses I engaged in to try to reposition him. Four days before my appointment he finally turned—and made us wait another two weeks for him. Then my water broke. The ambulance transported me to the birth clinic lying down. I unfortunately didn't have any contractions and only twenty-four hours to give birth, because a premature water breakage carries risk of infection. Because of my experience with my daughter's birth I asked for a contraction-promoting gel applied to the cervix. I wanted to give birth to my child actively this time, and so I chanted mantras and kept moving the whole time. Even as the pain increased I didn't lie down. Four hours later I gave birth to my son on a birthing stool while the doctor and midwife knelt on a mat in front of me. I was shaken and moved by the power of this spiritual experience. Even though my son had torn my already damaged pelvic-floor muscles, I didn't feel any pain, only unbelievable joy, pride, and humility.

Every birth is unique, but from my observation this life-altering event can often be enhanced if a woman starts preparing early for a self-determined birth. This preparation involves practicing fertility yoga and strengthening her trust in herself and her body.

To begin your practice you don't need much besides some determination and a certain degree of discipline. Gather a yoga mat, yoga cushion, light blanket, noncarbonated water to drink, and comfortable fitness clothes, ideally made of cotton. Prepare a place in your home for your practice so that you have to rearrange as little as possible each time you begin. If possible, engage in your practice at the same time each day in order to overcome the little voice inside of you that always tries to find excuses for avoiding your chosen discipline. Humans are creatures of habit—so create a habit! At the beginning you will probably be highly motivated to put what you learned from this book into practice. Next comes the disillusionment phase, however, which you will have to overcome with perseverance on your yoga mat. After that, your body will start craving the practice on its own. I recommend sticking it out for at least four weeks; after that it will get easier.

The exact nature of your practice depends on you. If you prefer completing a set of continuous poses, try the "Breath Exercises and Meditations for Emotional and Hormonal Balance" starting on page 104. If you have less time and would like to choose the poses yourself, pick a few from the fertility poses (at least four); men should practice all of the poses aimed specifically at them. Next, start adding the partner poses to your practice. Or only do the partner poses. It is better to do fewer poses regularly than many sporadically. After all, you are ultimately trying to stimulate your fertility and to energize your hormonal system; doing so will require some commitment. As I wrote at the beginning of this book, energy follows attention.

Concentration and dedication are far more important than perfection. Don't get upset if you're unable to master the positions at first, or if you're unable to sit or stretch very well. This will improve as time goes on, and the practice is still effective no matter your level of skill—simply do your best.

While other forms of yoga recommend using props like blocks, belts, and bands, I only recommend one: the high seat cushion (yoga or meditation cushion), which allows you to better relax your hips during meditation, breath exercises, or practice.

Take time for yourself, ideally thirty minutes to one hour daily, to concentrate on your fertility yoga practice. Turn off your phones, computer, and doorbell, and put on some soft, relaxing music.

Yoga Poses for Women

The following set of exercises are meant for women. The exercises focus on the second chakra, as the seat of sexual creativity, and the sixth chakra, as the center of hormonal balance. They let energy flow into the stomach and pelvis, ensure hormonal balance, and encourage female fertility. They encompass both static poses, held through a series of deep, long breaths (see page 104), and dynamic poses, which combine movement and faster breathing. Take a one- to two-minute break between poses, and, with your eyes closed, feel the effects they are having on your body and mind. Breathe slowly and consciously, and in a state of active awareness perceive what effect the respective poses are having on you—without judgment. You can practice all of the poses, or choose your favorites, practicing those regularly.

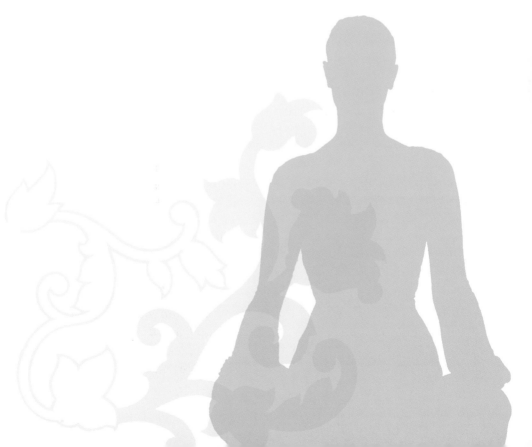

1. Breath Balancing Pose

This exercise balances your hormonal system and brings it into harmony with your central nervous system.

* Sit cross-legged (in the easy pose), keeping your spine straight. If needed, you can sit on a yoga cushion.

* Bend your arms, bringing your hands together in front of your heart. Lay your outstretched right hand over the left, so that both palms face your body, the fingers of your left hand pointing to the right, and the fingers of your right hand pointing to the left. Your hands and arms should be parallel to the ground.

* Press the tips of your thumbs together.

* Close your eyes almost all the way, leaving them open only a small sliver.

* Inhale deeply, and hold the breath in for ten seconds.

* Exhale completely and hold the breath out for ten seconds before taking another breath. In order to stimulate your central nervous system, it is important that you exhale completely.

* Concentrating on your breath, practice this exercise for three minutes.

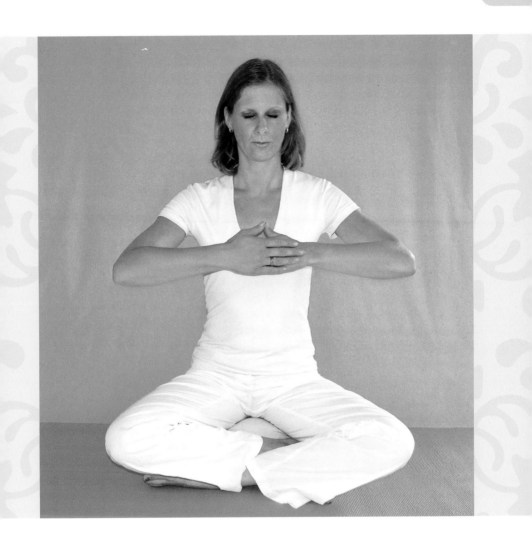

2. Bridge Pose

This exercise relaxes the lower body—particularly the ovaries, which hold psychological stress as tension. When practiced regularly, this exercise can lead to a regular menstrual cycle with reduced menstrual cramps. It also strengthens the sciatic nerve.

* Lie down on your back.
* Bend your knees and place your heels close to your buttocks.
* If you are able to, grab your ankles with your hands. If not, position your hands as close to your ankles as possible.
* While exhaling, lift your pelvis and raise your navel as high as possible.
* Hold the pose for two minutes while taking long, deep breaths.
* Slowly lower your back down to the floor, stretch out your legs, and relax.

Variation: In the dynamic version of this pose, take a deep, forceful breath while lifting your pelvis, then lower it back to the ground while exhaling.

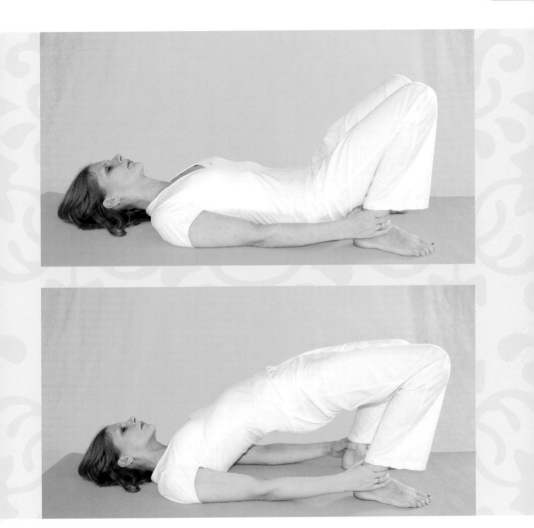

3. Venus Lock Pose

This exercise stimulates the ovaries, regulates the menstrual cycle, and eliminates digestive gas.

* Sit upright on the floor. Extend your left leg and either lay your right foot on your left thigh or bring the sole of your right foot to the inner side of your left thigh.

* Clasp your hands together behind your back. This hand pose is called the Venus lock.

* Bend your upper body forward, lowering your forehead toward your knee. At the same time, lift your locked arms upward, pulling your shoulder blades together.

* Hold this pose for two minutes.

* Switch legs and repeat.

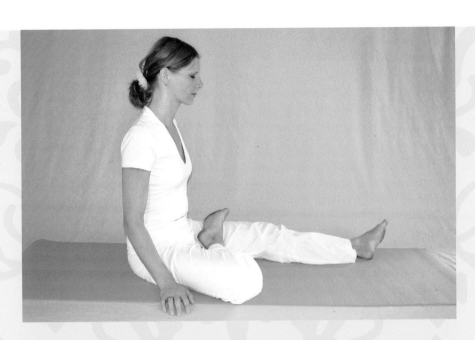

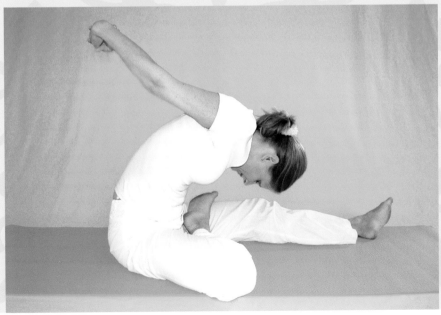

4. Mountain Pose and Standing Forward Bend

These two related poses balance the menstrual cycle and help alleviate PMS, which is characterized by physical discomfort, feelings of insecurity, and overly emotional behavioral right before the start of your period. These poses are also recommended for women experiencing difficulties during menopause. They stimulate fertility through their strong effect on the second chakra.

* Stand up straight. Your feet should be pointing slightly outwards, and your heels should be about hip width apart.

* Stretch your arms above your head with your palms facing forward. Link your thumbs and bring your upper arms close to your ears.

* Bend slightly backward while tightening your stomach and pelvic muscles. Hold this pose for two minutes while taking long, deep breaths.

* Next, start to slowly bend forward. If you're able to, lower your hands all the way to the floor while keeping your legs straight.

* Let your head hang down in a relaxed position, and inhale deeply.

* Holding the breath in, push your navel in and out using your stomach muscles, as many times as you are able to.

* Exhale completely and inhale again. Hold the breath in and repeat the pumping motion with your navel.

* Practice this for two minutes.

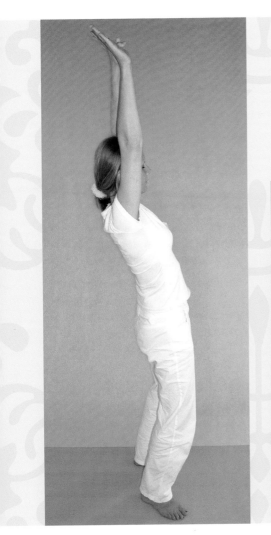

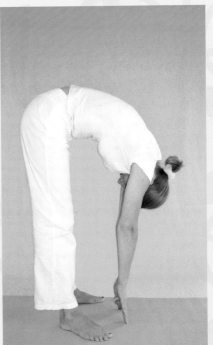

5. Butterfly Pose

This pose opens the hips and lower back and has a strengthening and harmonizing effect on the ovaries and pelvic region. It is recommended for menstrual cramps as well as in preparation for giving birth.

* Sitting on the ground, bring the soles of your feet together, pulling your heels as close as possible to your body.
* Keep your spine as straight as possible.
* Placing your hands around the balls of your feet, move your knees gently up and down for one minute, in order to relax your hips.
* While exhaling, bend your upper body forward and lift it up again, in one fluid movement.
* Sitting up straight, inhale, and while exhaling gently bend forward; then lift your upper body back up again.
* Repeat this sequence for one minute.
* Then, while maintaining your forward bend, move your feet a bit farther away from your body, and hold this pose for a few breaths.
* Send your healing, relaxing breath through your hips, pelvis, and reproductive organs.
* Upon exhaling, let go of all of the tension you are holding in these areas.

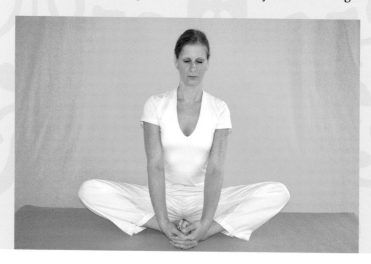

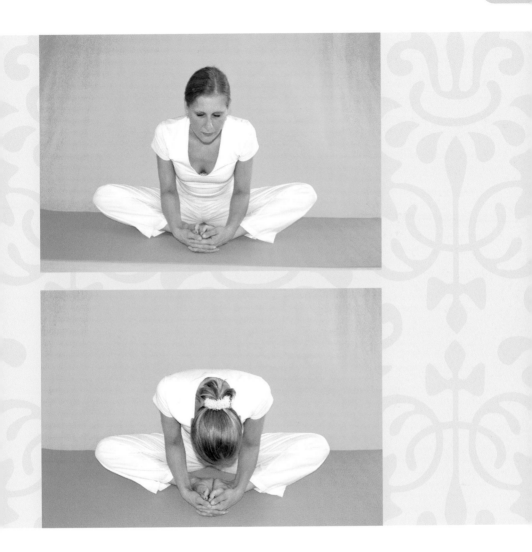

6. Plow Pose

A classic yoga pose, the plow has a stimulating effect on the hormone system and relieves strain on the stomach and reproductive organs. Inverted positions reverse the effect of gravity on the body, thereby relaxing the internal organs. If you are excessively overweight, this pose may be uncomfortable as it exerts a lot of pressure on the diaphragm. You should avoid inverted poses like the plow during menstruation, as they can cause cessation of or increased menstrual flow.

* Lie on your back with your arms resting near your body palms up.
* Bend your knees, bringing your feet toward your buttocks, with soles of the feet resting on the floor.
* While tightening your pelvic and stomach muscles, lift your legs and buttocks while supporting your hips and lower back with your hands.
* Extend your legs over your head. At the same time, roll onto your upper back and shoulders for support so that your chin is close to your chest.
* Lower your feet to the floor behind your head. If able, keep your legs fully extended while doing this. If this is too difficult, place a cushion or a rolled up blanket behind your head for your feet to rest on, or prop your feet against a wall behind you.

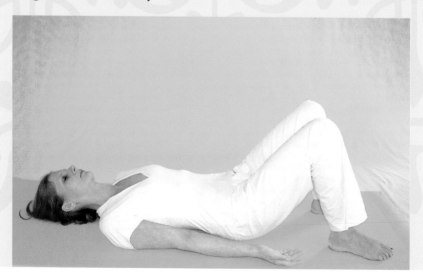

* If you are feeling secure and confident in this position, place your hands on the floor next to your body, palms down.

* Relax and spend two minutes taking long, deep breaths.

* Reposition your hands to support your lower back once again, bend your legs, and roll slowly back onto the ground, one vertebra at a time.

* Take a minute to rest with your legs fully extended.

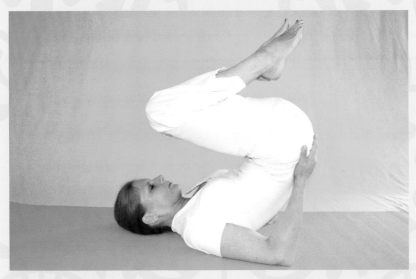

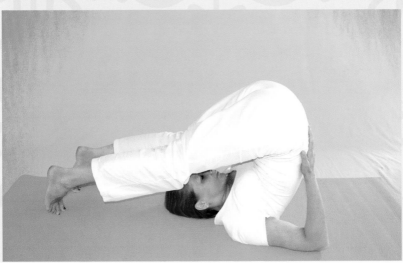

7. Bow Pose

The bow pose regulates the female hormone system and promotes emotional stability. It also intensifies blood circulation to the pelvic and internal organs.

* Lie on your stomach with your legs spread slightly apart, arms close to your body, and forehead gently resting on the floor.
* Bend your knees, bringing your feet close to your buttocks, and take hold of your ankles with your hands.
* Inhale deeply and pull your body upward. In so doing, lift your chest and upper thighs off the ground with your arms extended.
* Breathe deeply and steadily.
* Hold this position for one to two minutes, or as long as you're able.

Variation: In the dynamic version of this pose, pull your body up while inhaling, and let it fall gently back to the ground upon exhaling.

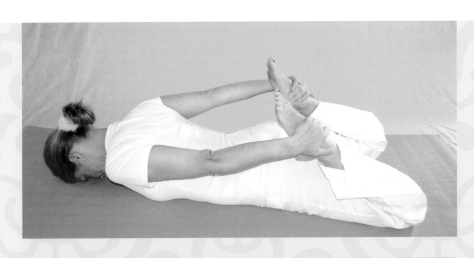

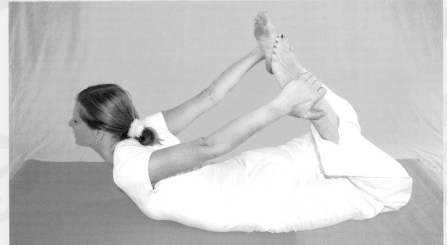

8. Reclining Hero Pose

This pose revitalizes and rejuvenates the reproductive organs and stimulates the hormone system. It opens the hips and pelvis.

* From a kneeling position, slowly lower your buttocks to the ground between your heels.
* Placing your hands on the floor behind your back for support, slowly lean back.
* Bend your arms and lower your weight onto your elbows.
* If you are able, slowly lean back even farther until you are lying on the ground.
* Relax your shoulders, extend your arms alongside your torso, palms up, and breathe into your chest and hips.
* Remain in this position for two minutes, and then raise yourself back up onto your elbows while tightening your stomach and pelvic muscles. Keeping your muscles taut, return to a sitting position.
* Extend your legs in front of you, and lean gently forward, relaxing your neck for a few breaths.

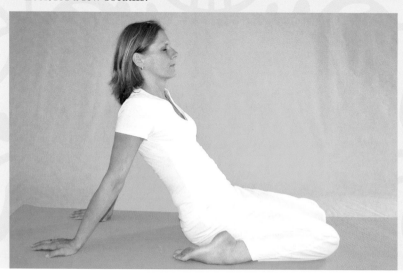

Variation: If this pose puts too much pressure on your thighs, knees, and lower back, sit cross-legged and, supporting your body with your hands behind you, lean back slowly until you are lying on the floor.

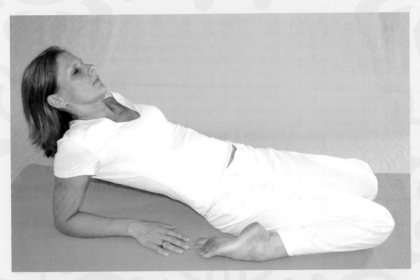

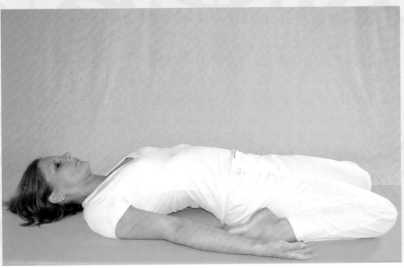

9. Wheel Pose

The wheel is an advanced, challenging pose. You should only integrate it into your routine once you feel confident in the bridge pose and trust the strength of your arms. You should avoid this pose if you have high blood pressure. The wheel pose increases the flexibility of the spine and strengthens the muscles in the stomach, legs, and arms. As the head hangs backward and down in this pose, it draws energy to the brain and stimulates the hypothalamus and pituitary glands, both of which significantly regulate your hormone system. Because everything is "turned on its head" in this inverted pose, it can also help you view your own situation in a new light.

- Lie on your back, with your knees bent and feet on the ground.
- While exhaling, lift yourself into the bridge pose, and place your hands on the ground behind your shoulders, with your fingers pointing towards your shoulders.
- Push yourself up higher and lift your shoulders from the ground until only the top of your head is touching the ground.
- Then lift your head from the ground by straightening your arms and raising your hips and stomach towards the ceiling.
- Your feet should be turned slightly outward while your hands should be pointed slightly inwards.
- Hold this pose for several breaths, then slowly and carefully lower your head, your upper body, and then the rest of your torso.
- Stretch out your legs and take a few moments to rest.
- Feel the flow of energy through your body.

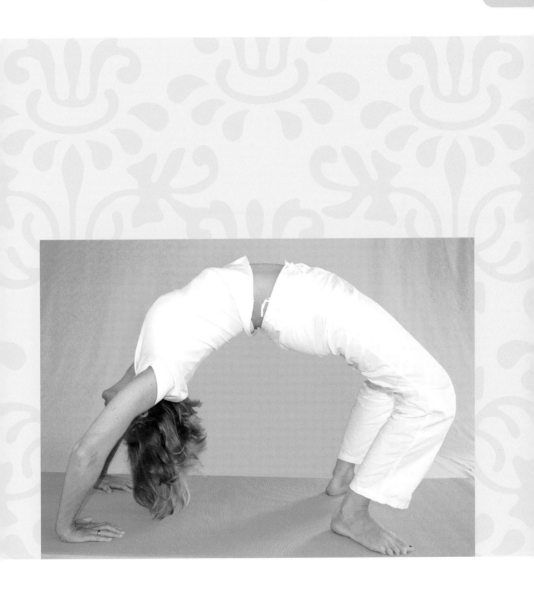

Yoga Poses for Men

As already mentioned, approximately half of fertility problems are attributed to the male partner. With this special program, male fertility can be increased. The regular practice of these poses improves sperm quality and quantity as well as sexual potency.

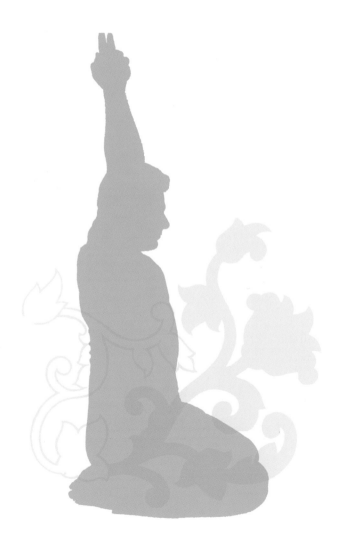

1. Archer Pose

The archer pose strengthens masculine potency and the nervous system. It helps promote a calm, centered mind able to meet the challenges of the everyday.

* Stand with your legs straight and far apart, feet parallel to one another.

* Rotate your right foot outward so that it is perpendicular to your left foot. Turn your head in the same direction as your right foot.

* Bend your right knee so that it is positioned directly over your toes.

* Lift your right arm to shoulder height in front of you, and make a fist with your thumb extended and pointing toward the ceiling.

* With your left hand, grip toward your right wrist and pull back your imaginary bow.

* Position your left fist at the height of your left armpit, as if you were holding a taught bow. Both arms should be in line with each other.

* Gaze toward the fingernail of your right thumb, and simultaneously toward an imaginary point in the distance.

* Breathe slowly and calmly. Hold this pose for two minutes.

* To end, inhale deeply and hold the breath in while fixating on your goal. Fire your arrow and relax.

* Change sides and repeat.

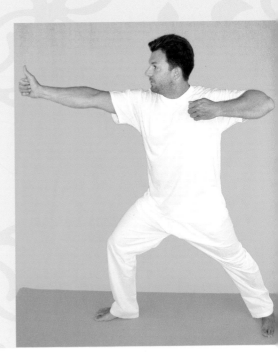

2. Frog Pose

In ancient India, growing boys had to regularly practice the frog. They were only considered ready to marry when they could perform one hundred at a time. This pose strengthens the first and second chakras, trains the thigh muscles, and stretches the back of the legs. It also stimulates circulation and improves sperm production.

* Crouch on the balls of your feet with your heels touching each other and knees spread wide.
* Place the tips of your fingers on the ground between your legs, and hold your upper body upright.
* Your eyes should be open.
* Inhale vigorously, lift your buttocks up, and straighten your legs. If possible, your hands or fingertips should still touch the ground.
* While exhaling, return to your initial position.
* Repeat for two minutes, taking vigorous breaths.
* To end, straighten your legs again, release your hands from the ground, and slowly return, vertebra by vertebra, to a standing position.

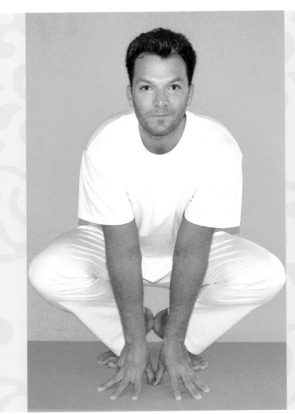
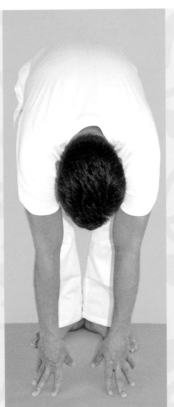

3. Chair Pose

The chair pose has a powerful strengthening effect on the first, second, and third chakras. It strengthens the thigh muscles and opens the hips. It also increases circulation and energy flow to the pelvic and reproductive organs.

* Stand with your feet placed shoulder width apart, and turn them slightly outwards.

* Inhale deeply and bend your knees so that your weight is concentrated on your heels rather than on the balls of your feet. Lower your buttocks to knee level, thighs parallel to the ground.

* Reach your hands through the inside of your legs and grab your heels. Your head, spine, and tailbone should form a line parallel to the ground.

* Hold this position for one minute, taking long, deep breaths.

* Release your hands, positioning them in front of you on the ground, and straighten your legs.

* Hold this position for a few breaths, and while exhaling slowly return to a standing position.

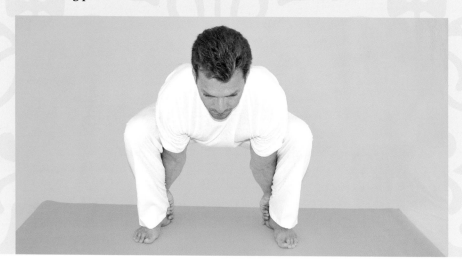

4. Sat Kriya

This exercise energizes all of the chakras and brings energy from the base of the spine into the center of higher consciousness. It strengthens the stomach and pelvic muscles and straightens the spine. It also fortifies the male reproductive organs, thereby preventing impotence. This powerful exercise should be practiced daily.

* Sit on your heels or cross-legged (the easy pose). You can use a yoga cushion if needed.

* Straighten your arms above your head and interlock your fingers so that your forefingers are pointed upwards, and your thumbs are crossed over one another.

* Your upper arms should be close to your ears. Relax your shoulders.

* Close your eyes and focus your concentration on the point between your eyebrows.

* Vocalize a loud "SSSAT," and simultaneously pull your stomach, diaphragm, and testicles quickly and energetically into your body.

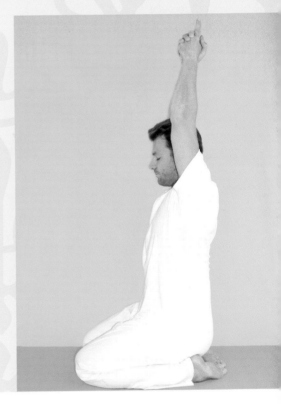

* Now vocalize "NAAAM," and relax your muscles.

* Repeat the mantras in a steady, moderate tempo while moving your stomach forward and back. Tense your stomach and pelvic muscles respectively, and then relax them again.

* Practice this for three minutes. Then inhale once more, hold your breath, and tense all of your internal muscles. Imagine that you're concentrating all of your energy in your spine and drawing it upward.

* Exhale and let your arms fall back down by your sides.

* Continue to imagine this energy for a few more breaths.

Yoga Poses for Couples

The following exercises should be practiced together. They strengthen your connection as a couple and as future parents and stimulate creativity, sensuality, and reproductive capability.

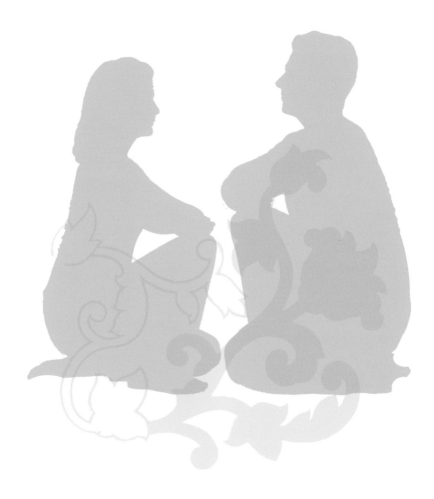

1. "I Am You"

This exercise stimulates the sexual glands and regulates the interplay between pancreas, adrenal glands, and kidneys. It cleanses the blood and promotes the flow of energy through the body's main energy highway, the spine. It thereby helps to prevent heart problems and promotes a long lifespan.

* Position yourselves on the floor, facing each other.

* Sit upright on your left heel so that it presses against your perineum.

* Position your right leg so that your knee is close to your chest.

* Bend your arms, and place your left hand on your knee and your right hand on top of your left, thumbs touching. Hold your arms parallel to the ground.

* Close your eyes and look within yourself.

* Take four loud, audible breaths of equal length. While doing this, think, "Ong Ong Ong Ong."

* Exhale in four loud breaths while thinking, "Sohung Sohung Sohung Sohung." The mantra "Ong Sohung" means "I am you" and also "We are one."

* Practice this for five minutes.

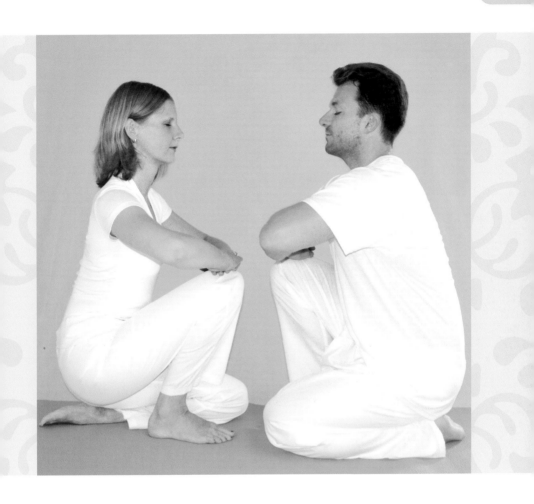

2. The Crow

This exercise opens the pelvis and stretches the thighs. Energetically, the crow affects the first and second chakras, the centers of connection with the earth, sexuality, and vitality. It also strengthens your connection with each other and promotes mutual trust.

* Stand facing each other with your feet hip width apart.

* Take each other's hands so that the male partner's palms face upward and the female partner's palms face downward.

* Look your partner steadily and lovingly in the eyes.

* Inhale deeply together, and upon exhaling, bend your knees. The soles of your feet should stay flat on the ground, and your buttocks should bend as low as possible.

* Slowly lean back, finding the point where you balance each other. You are each supporting both your partner and yourself.

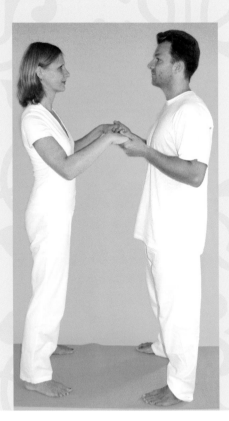

✳ Remain in this position, holding both hand and eye contact and taking long, deep breaths.

✳ After two minutes, inhale again deeply, bend your arms, and while exhaling stand up together.

✳ Release your hands and shake out your arms and legs.

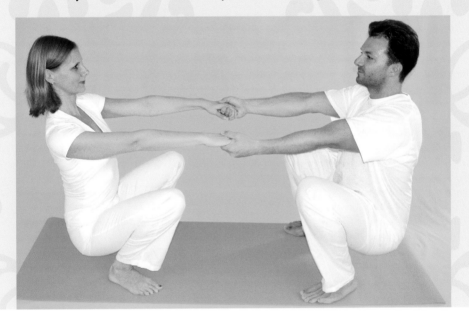

3. The Cogged Wheel

This exercise stimulates both fertility and life energy by increasing the flexibility of the spine. It simultaneously promotes a feeling of empathy for your partner, since your movements have to be in sync with one another's in order for the pose to be pleasant for both partners.

✳ Sit on the ground back to back.

✳ Initiate contact with your partner. Feel his or her warmth, weight, and pure presence.

✳ Breathe calmly and deeply, finding a common rhythm for your breath.

✳ While exhaling, the female partner bends forward while the male partner simultaneously leans back.

✳ With the next inhalation switch roles, with the female partner leaning on her partner's back, relaxed.

✳ Imagine that your vertebrae are like cogs on a wheel that interlock with one another.

✳ Continue this movement back and forth for three minutes.

✳ Then return to the middle position, inhaling and sensing your backs simultaneously supporting one another.

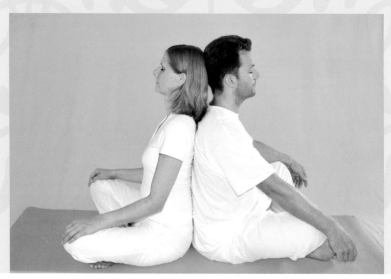

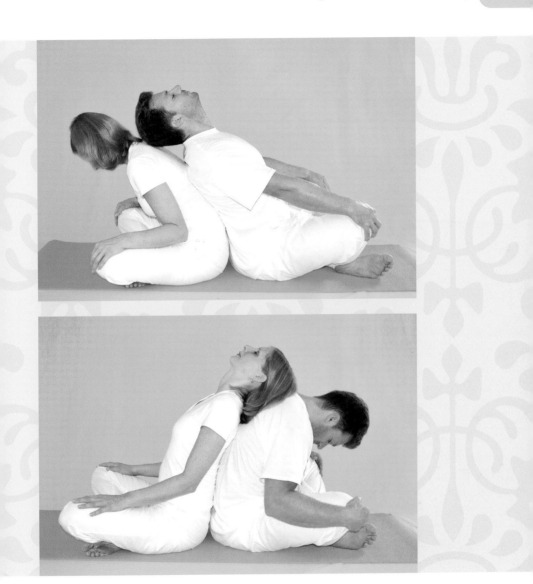

Series of Exercises for Hormonal Balance

The pituitary gland is the primary organ that controls hormonal balance. It is yogically connected with the third eye—also called the sixth chakra—the home of your sixth sense, which sharpens your awareness of the other five senses. A harmoniously functioning sixth chakra is evidenced through holistic thoughts and a sense of trust in your own intuition. The following series of exercises is for the pituitary gland. When practiced regularly it promotes a calm and centered mind that employs the power of imagination, and a hormonal balance in the body that is the basic component of fertility. The exercises stimulate the thyroid and parathyroid glands and promote a strong central nervous system.

With the fertility exercises described earlier I encouraged you to pick and choose your favorite poses; by contrast, with this series it is important to practice each exercise in its proper order in order to maximize its full energetic effect. The series is meant for both men and women—and it is always nice to practice them together.

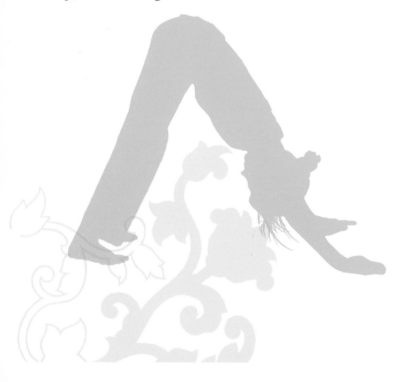

1. Forward Lunge Pose

* Bend your left knee and place it with your foot flat on the ground. Extend your right leg behind you, and support yourself by placing your hands on either side of your left foot on the floor.

* Hold your head as high as possible and inclined slightly backwards.

* Take long, deep breaths for one minute.

* Next, practice the breath of fire for two minutes: Take fast, rhythmic breaths, pulling your navel inward upon exhaling.

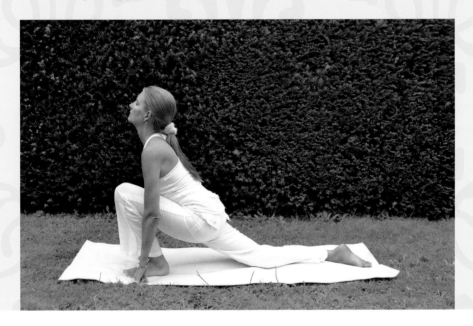

2. Pose for the Pituitary Gland and Ovaries

✳ From the last position, lower your left knee to the ground and lean forward until your whole body is resting on your left thigh.

✳ Lower your forehead to the floor and extend your right leg as far back as possible. Extend your arms along your sides, with your palms facing up.

✳ Hold this position for three minutes while taking long, deep breaths.

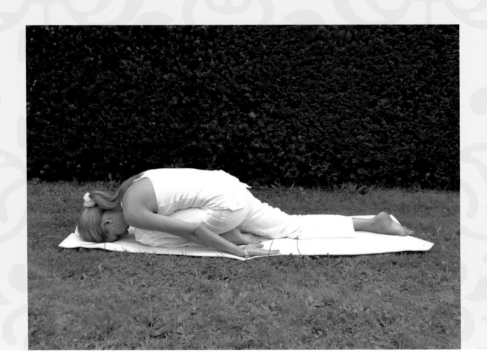

3./4. Repeat

✳ Repeat exercises 1 and 2, changing sides.

5. Forward Bend Pose

✳ Stand up, placing your feet hip width apart.

✳ Lift your arms up, palms facing upward.

✳ Bend forward and touch the ground with your palms or fingertips.

✳ Hold this position for three minutes while taking long, deep breaths.

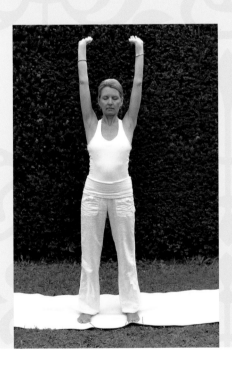
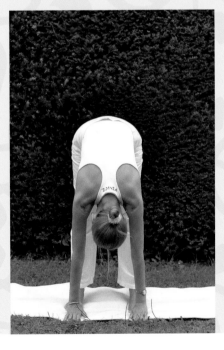

6. "Ego Destroyer" Pose

* Return to a standing position and raise your arms above your head, hands closed in fists and thumbs extended to point toward each other. Arms should be at a sixty-degree angle to one another.

* Push through your elbows and breathe deeply for three minutes.

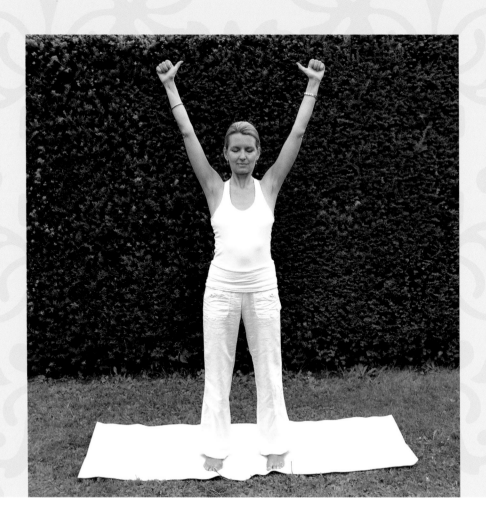

7. Downward-Facing Dog Pose

* Come down to the floor on your hands and knees.
* Lift your pelvis and straighten your arms and legs until your body forms a triangle. Your head and neck should be relaxed.
* Straighten your back by pressing your breastbone toward the floor.
* Try to lower your heels to the floor. If that is not possible with your legs fully extended, bend your knees slightly.
* Hold this position for three minutes, keeping your weight evenly distributed between hands and feet.

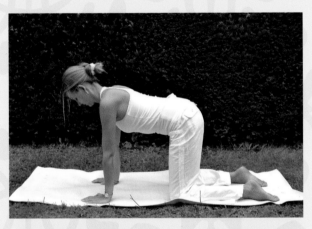

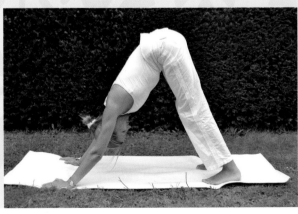

8. Cobra Pose

❋ Lie down on your stomach and relax for one minute.

❋ Bring your heels close to one another and place your hands on the floor next to your shoulders.

❋ Lift your upper body off of the floor and tilt your head and neck back.

❋ Take long, deep breaths for one minute.

❋ For two minutes, turn your head to the left upon inhaling, and to the right upon exhaling.

❋ To conclude, exhale and tense your stomach and pelvic muscles. Roll slowly down to the floor and relax for a few breaths.

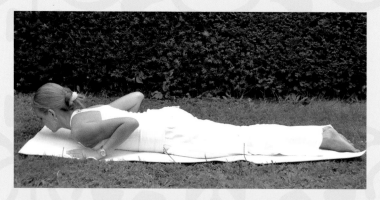

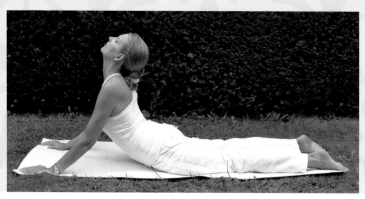

9. Flower Pose

✳ Sit on your heels with your knees slightly apart.

✳ Inhale and lift yourself into a knee stand. Lift your arms toward the sky, angled outward a bit, like a flower greeting the sun.

✳ Exhale and lower your forehead to the floor, placing your hands palms down in front of your knees. Forearms should be resting on the floor.

✳ Repeat the movement sequence in rhythm with your breath for three minutes.

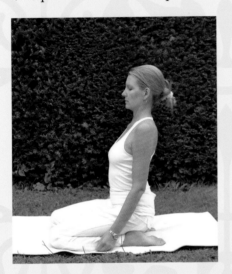
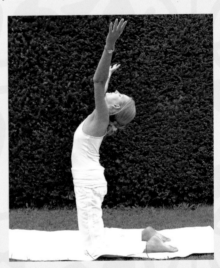
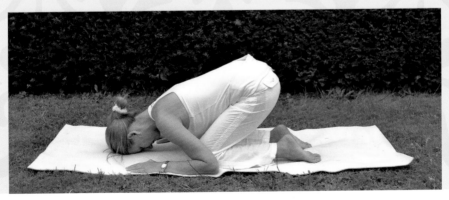

10. Yoga Mudra Pose

✳ Sit back on your heels, with your knees touching.

✳ Extend your hands behind your back and interlace your fingers.

✳ Lower your forehead to the floor and lift your straightened arms behind you as high as possible.

✳ Hold this position, breathing deeply for three minutes.

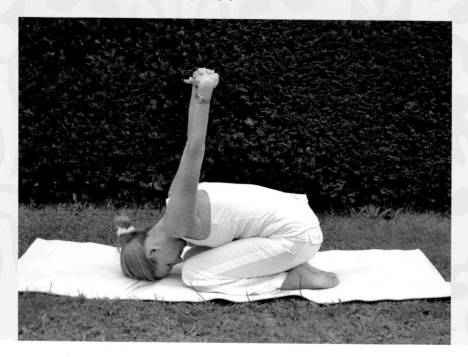

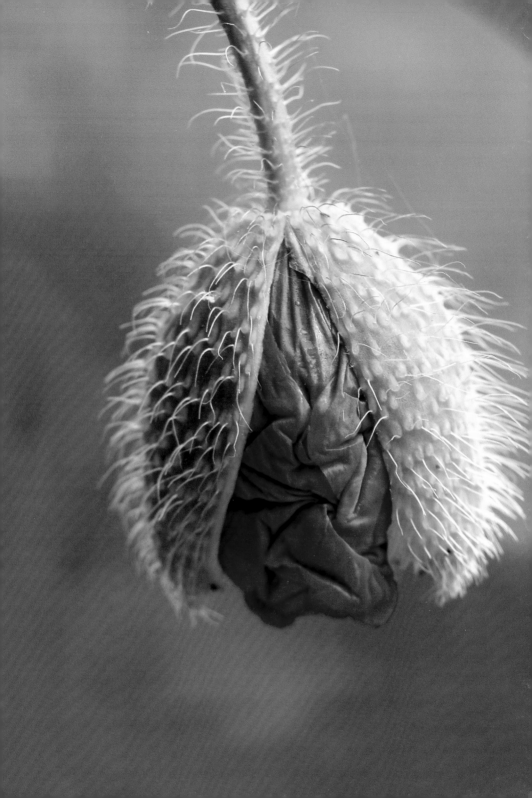

CHAPTER 4

BREATH EXERCISES AND MEDITATIONS FOR EMOTIONAL AND HORMONAL BALANCE

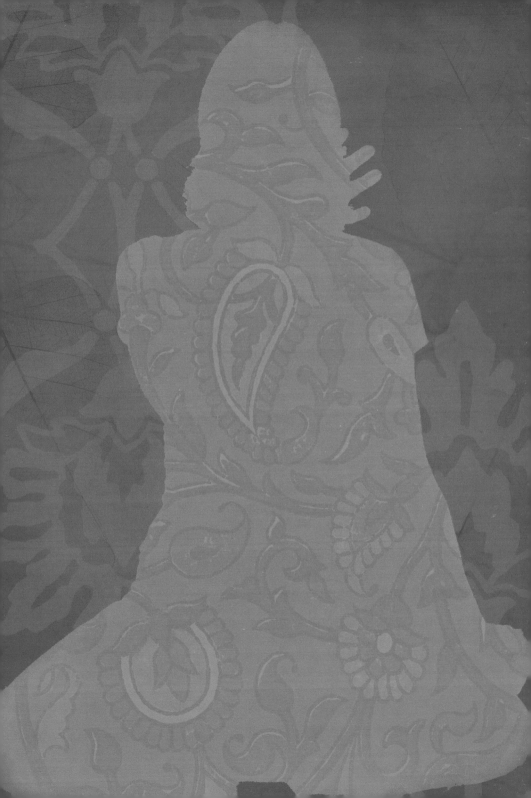

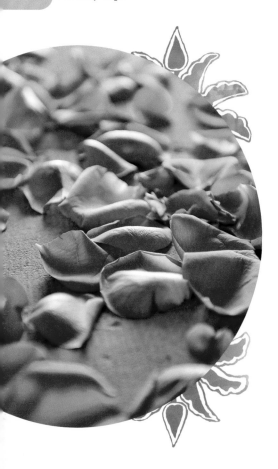

Breath and Relaxation

We saw earlier in the book how stress and emotional strain can negatively affect a woman's fertility. Male fertility is also negatively impacted by chronic stress. Deep breathing can help to resolve and counter this stress. Nothing affects your psychological well-being and mood as much as your breath. Breathing is a semiautonomic process—we all breathe automatically from birth until death, but the quality of breath varies and can be deliberately altered. We normally breathe between fifteen and twenty times per minute. The ancient yogis recommended, however, that we slow our breathing to between five and seven breaths per minute. According to oral tradition, the length of each life is limited by a predetermined number of breaths that individual will take. If one uses their breath sparingly, they theoretically will live longer. Breathing slowly and deeply has an almost immediate relaxing and calming effect on the body. As my yoga teacher says, "Now that you know this, all your problems will be solved." If only it were so simple. The secret is to stick with the practice of slow and deep breathing and remember to return to it in critical situations.

In yoga there are several breath exercises, called *pranayama*, that promote varying energetic effects. Mastering your breath has a positive effect not only on your mood and current emotional state but also on your physical body by helping to release deep-seated tension. The yoga breath is usually a purely nasal breath. (There are a few exceptions that have specific energetic effects.) That means, unlike with other physical practices, in yoga one breathes exclusively in and out of the nose. Because the nasal passages run along the base of the skull, breathing through the nose stimulates the pituitary gland, which primarily controls hormone balance. If you were able to breathe throughout the day as you are encouraged to breathe during yoga practice, all of your stress and tension would simply fall away. Try to avoid returning to your familiar patterns of thinking and behavior when the exercise is over.

Taking long, deep breaths improves the oxygen supply to the entire body, down to the cellular level. It also permanently stimulates metabolism and other bodily systems, including the lymphatic, hormonal, and circulatory systems. It allows you to develop a greater sense of your body and its complex, inner processes that are all striving toward a harmonious balance. Breathing deeply and regularly thus stimulates your powers of self-healing and improves your feelings of well-being on a larger, holistic level.

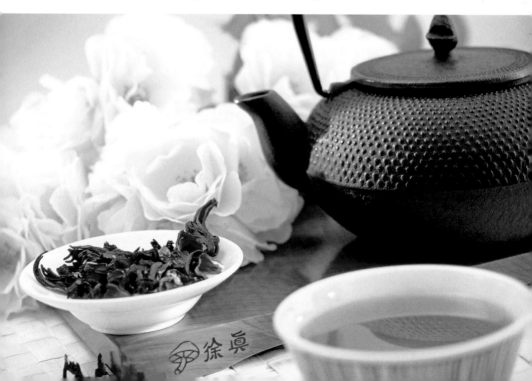

1. Deep Stomach Breathing

When you take long, deep breaths you are consciously, slowly, and completely breathing "into your stomach." This, of course, is physiologically impossible; it is another way of saying that your stomach muscles should be completely relaxed. When you inhale, your abdominal wall should bulge outward, so that your diaphragm, your largest breath-related muscle, has room to relax downward. In yoga, the breath is fundamental for all meditation, breath, and yoga practices, and should therefore be practiced regularly so that you become accustomed to this conscious method of breathing.

✳ Sit down on the floor, a pillow, or a chair—the important thing is that you're comfortable. Relax your legs, hips, and shoulders. Rest your hands lightly on your knees, palms down.

✳ Straighten your spine, imagining a thread attached to the top of your head that is pulling your spine tall without any exertion on your part.

✳ Close your eyes and focus your attention inward.

✳ Relax your jaw, keeping it slack, with your teeth slightly apart.

✳ Your tongue should lie in a relaxed state, your lips touching each other softly.

✳ Begin to slowly inhale through your nose, pressing your tongue lightly against your upper palate.

✳ Consciously push out your stomach, expanding your ribs while your breath flows fully inward.

✳ Take a moment to experience the fullness of your complete inhalation—but don't force yourself to hold the air in uncomfortably—before you slowly let the breath completely flow out through your nose.

✳ While exhaling, let your stomach relax. If you'd like, you can actively pull your stomach in at the end, to make sure the last bit of breath is pushed out.

✳ Take a moment to feel the emptiness of your full exhalation before you inhale once again.

* Each breath you take flows ever deeper and increases your connection with your innermost being, your essential core, your "true self" that lies hidden under the layers of the everyday.

* Try to produce a light rustling sound with your breath, like the sound of the sea.

* Practice this breathing technique for five minutes every day. Observe how you feel after the breath exercise.

* Once you are familiar with this style of breathing, visualize a healing light. For example, while inhaling imagine a warm, orange-colored light flowing into your reproductive organs, warming, stimulating, and healing them.

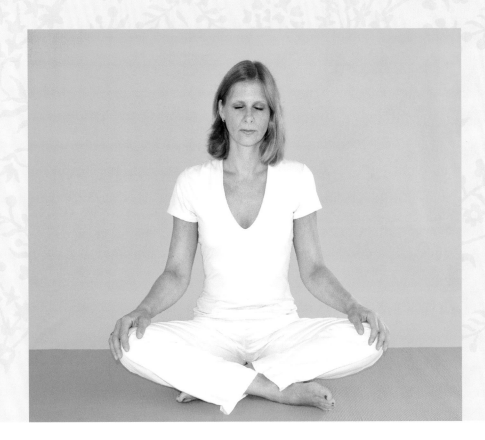

2. The Fourth Breath

A simple pattern of breath helps you stay grounded and focus upon yourself in any given situation. You can use it at any time—while walking, standing, or lying down—whenever you want to calm down and connect with your center. The fourth breath is especially useful in stressful situations, such as during doctor's appointments or when you're upset.

* Inhale slowly and consciously, as described for the deep stomach breath, while counting inwardly from one to four.

* Hold the breath in for four slow counts.

* Exhale at the same tempo while counting to four.

* Hold the breath out, thinking, "one—two—three—four."

* All four breath phases should be the same length: four counts of whatever rhythm you determine is best for you.

3. The Fundamental Breath Series

This breath series helps resolve psychological blockages, feelings of guilt, and fear of failure. It also supports hormonal balance and thus fertility. The amazing effects that concentrating on your third eye can have on your hormone system have yet to be imagined. The fundamental breath series gives you a quick energy boost, increases your clarity, and promotes feelings of balance and stability. It allows you to recognize your relationship with your breath and observe the differences between emotions and thoughts that every breath form brings up.

Even though breathing is the most natural thing in the world, conscious breathing can be quite challenging. As soon as you consciously alter your breath, you break the normal emotional and attentive patterns that underlie your physical and mental habits, beginning to resolve them. During this process it is possible that you will find yourself losing concentration. When you continue, however, you will gain a new feeling of lightness and the ability to better control your mind.

As a beginner start with shorter times, increasing them gradually over time.

Base Pose

✳ Sit cross-legged (in the easy pose) or in another upright sitting position that you are able to hold for at least fifteen minutes. If necessary, use a yoga cushion for sitting.

✳ Close your eyes and roll them gently upwards. Concentrate your gaze inwardly on your third eye, located at the bridge of your nose where your eyebrows come together.

Left-Side Breath (photo above right)

✳ Position your left hand in what is called the *gyan mudra*, with the tips of your thumb and forefinger touching. Your left arm should be extended, with your wrist resting on your left knee.

✳ Lift your right hand and press the inside of your thumb gently on your right nostril to close it, or place the tip of your thumb on the underside of your nostril. The other fingers should point upward like antennas.

✳ Take long, deep breaths, in and out, through your left nostril.

✳ Continue to breathe like this for three minutes.

✳ Take one more deep breath and hold it for ten to thirty seconds; then exhale and relax.

Right-Side Breath (photo below right)

✳ Lay your right hand in the gyan mudra on your right knee.

✳ Lift your left hand and softly close your left nostril with your thumb. The other fingers should be outstretched and pointing upward like antennas.

✳ Inhale and exhale deeply and slowly through your right nostril.

✳ Continue to breathe like this for three minutes.

✳ Take one more deep breath and hold it for ten to thirty seconds; then exhale and relax.

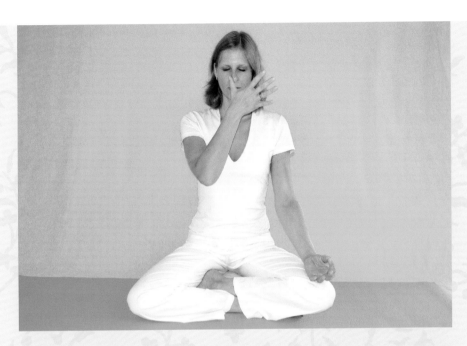

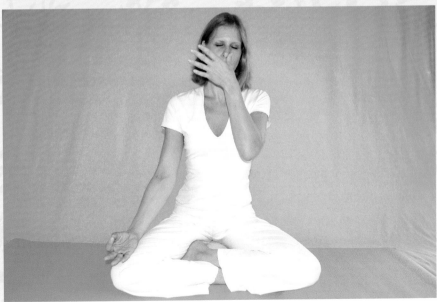

Alternating Breath Left/Right

❋ Stay in a seated position. Lay your left hand in the gyan mudra on your left knee.

❋ Close your right nostril with your right thumb and inhale deeply through your left nostril.

❋ Then press your left nostril closed with your right forefinger and open your right nostril at the same time, exhaling completely through your right nostril.

❋ Change fingers and inhale through your left nostril.

❋ Continue this alternate breathing—inhaling through your left nostril, exhaling through your right—for two to three minutes.

❋ To conclude, inhale deeply and hold the breath for ten to thirty seconds, then exhale and relax.

❋ Repeat the sequence with the other side, inhaling through your right nostril and exhaling through your left. Your right hand should be relaxed, resting in the gyan mudra on your right knee, as you close your nostrils alternately with your left thumb and forefinger.

Breath of Fire

❋ Remain in a seated position and lay both of your hands in the gyan mudra on your knees.

❋ Inhale quickly and powerfully through your nose while pushing your stomach outward (photo above right).

❋ Exhale forcefully while pulling your navel inward (photo lower right).

❋ Find a consistent rhythm for your breath, with each inhale and exhale lasting approximately one second. Emphasize your exhalations to avoid feeling light-headed.

❋ Continue this sequence for two to seven minutes. If necessary, take short breaks and breathe in a relaxed manner for a few breaths.

❋ To conclude, inhale once more and hold the breath for ten to sixty seconds. Observe how energy is circulating through your body.

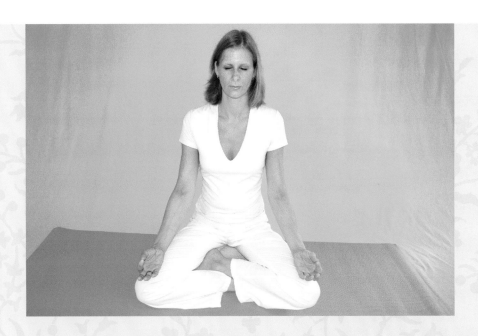

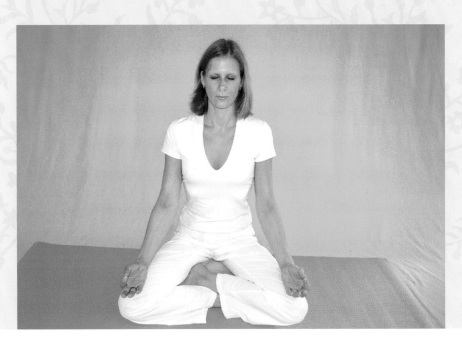

Meditation

❋ Relax and focus your concentration for one to three minutes on the natural flow of your breath, your river of energy. Observe how your mind and emotions have changed.

❋ Meditate for three to ten minutes on your "true self," thinking on "SAAAT" (truth) while inhaling and on "NAAAM" (identity) while exhaling. Clear your mind of all thoughts and listen to the silence within you.

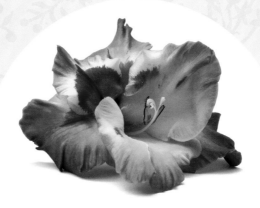

Meditations for Fertility Problems

What are fertility problems and why do they arise? Or, "Why do they have to happen to me/us, when everyone else seems to be having no problems having children?" This is a question that bothers many couples who are hoping for a baby, and one they seem to come back to again and again.

Sometimes there is no medical explanation for why a couple has trouble getting pregnant. They can only wait it out and simply let things run their course. The following two meditations are particularly helpful during this waiting period.

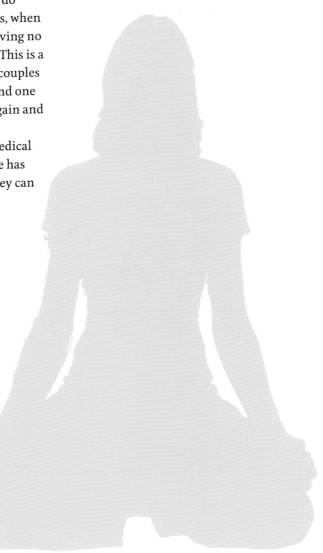

1. Meditation for a Tranquil Heart

The meditation for a tranquil heart helps you to come to terms with your current situation, and to become fully present in the here and now. Emotionally, the meditation leads to greater awareness of your relationship to both yourself and others. And when psychological blockages are resolved, it often leads to the desired pregnancy.

This meditation is perfect for beginners. It promotes an awareness of the breath and strengthens the lungs and heart. During this mediation the left hand rests on the heart, the natural seat of prana, or life energy. It induces a deep inner stillness. The right hand, which stands for action and analysis, is held in a receptive mudra in the position of peace. The whole posture promotes a feeling of stillness and serenity, and calms the life energy in your heart center.

* Sit cross-legged on the floor or on a hard cushion, straighten your spine, and find a relaxed sitting position.
* Close your eyes.
* Lay the palm of your left hand on your heart center, with your fingers pointing toward the right.
* Bring the thumb and forefinger of your right hand together into the gyan mudra—connect your ego (thumb) with wisdom (forefinger).
* Lift your right hand to the side as if you were swearing an oath. The palm should be facing forward, the fingers stretched upward.
* Concentrate on the flow of your breath. Consciously regulate each phase of your breath. Inhale slowly and deeply through both nostrils, expand your chest, push your stomach outward, and hold the breath in as long as possible. Then exhale slowly, steadily, and completely, letting your stomach relax, and hold the breath out.

* *Warning:* Don't hold your breath so long that you end up gasping for air or feeling under pressure when you take your next breath. Don't get over-ambitious—accept your personal boundaries.

* Meditate in this manner for three to eleven minutes. As you become more advanced, the meditation can be extended to thirty-one minutes; it then becomes a challenging exercise in concentration and regeneration.

* To end the exercise, inhale and exhale normally three times and then relax.

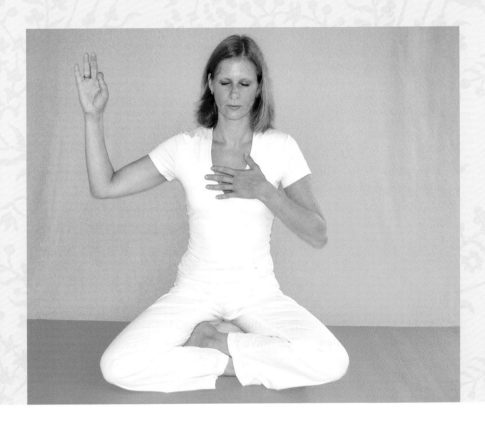

2. Meditation for the Endocrine (Hormonal) System

This meditation should be practiced for at least forty consecutive days in order to revitalize your entire endocrine system and bring it into balance. It is effective as a "survival strategy," a meditation technique meant especially for dealing with the stress and pressures of our time. It is extraordinarily relaxing. According to yogic knowledge, the pituitary gland controls the functioning of the sexual glands, hormone release, and sexual sensation. This meditation uses breath to affect the main controlling gland of the body, thereby revitalizing the entire hormonal system.

* Sit in an upright position on the floor. If necessary, sit on a cushion.

* Hold your arms to the side, bend your elbows, and lay your right hand over your left. Your palms should be facing your body at about heart level. Your left thumb should lie in the middle of your right palm, with the right thumb crossing the left.

* Close your eyes until you can only see a small sliver of light. It is also okay if your eyes are completely closed during the meditation.

* Inhale deeply, and while exhaling sing the mantra "SAAAT NAM." The syllable "SAT" should be thirty-five times as long as the syllable "NAM."

* Meditate in this way for eleven minutes. Then inhale and exhale deeply a few times, open your eyes, and shake out your hands.

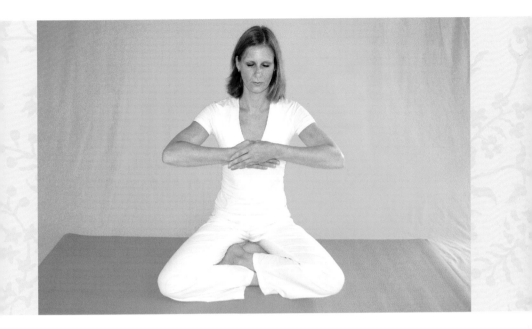

More Helpful Meditations for Conceiving a Child

As with everything else in life, it is only possible to bear children for a limited time. There are four big phases of life: childhood and youth, in which you grow and mature; early adulthood, in which you find your place in the world and establish a family; middle age, in which you see your children grow and venture out into the world; and old age, in which you gain wisdom and prepare yourself to leave the world.

Not everyone, of course, must fulfill the biological laws of reproduction. In today's world you can choose not to have children and use the energy you would have otherwise invested in a family for other pursuits. Women and couples with a strong desire to have children often get energetically stuck in a stage of unfulfilled yearning, blocking themselves instead of letting go and simply trusting that everything happens for a reason—that a life without children can also be fulfilling and filled with meaning.

When you succeed in letting go you may find yourself inspired with a new perspective on life and what it has to offer. Sometimes the work of wishing for a child can lead to resolving deep-seated blockages so that even the impossible can become possible. In my work with pregnant women I have known a few who had given up hope of conceiving a child and adopted a baby, only to become pregnant and give birth to a healthy child later on, much to the surprise of the doctors who had diagnosed them with infertility.

1. Meditation for Harmonization

Kirtan Kriya, the meditation for harmonization, symbolizes the cycle of creation. From infinity emerges life and individual existence, and from life emerges death as an aspect of transformation into another state of existence. From death emerges the rebirth of the consciousness into human existence through its empathy and connectedness.

The Kirtan Kriya is one of the fundamental meditations of kundalini yoga. When you practice it on a regular basis, it brings your hormones into balance, stimulates your self-healing powers, and strengthens your hormonal system.

✳ Sit on the floor with legs crossed and back straight. If necessary, sit on a cushion.

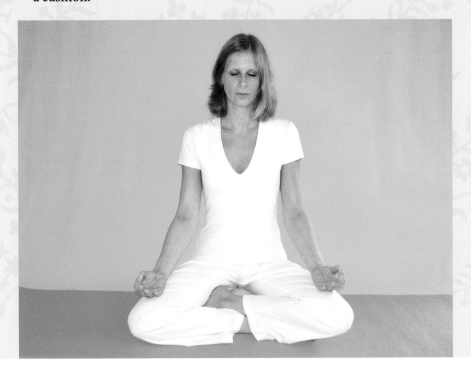

✻ Meditate while concentrating on your third eye and singing, "SA, TA, NA, MA," the five primary sounds (S, T, N, M, A), also known as "Panj Shabad."

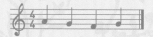

"SA" signifies infinity, the cosmos, and new beginnings, "TA" life and existence, "NA" death, and "MA" rebirth. Chanting, which is the monotone singing of mantras, these five sounds is the original "core form" of the mantra "SAT NAM." Each repetition of the mantra should last around four seconds.

✻ While chanting, lay your hands, palms facing up, on your knees. With every syllable, bring the tip of one finger together with the tip of your thumb. Each time you form a circle with your thumb and another finger, you create a mudra and thereby stimulate your consciousness. See the table below for a brief explanation of each mudra and the various energies and heavenly bodies it is associated with.

FINGER	NAME	PLANET/STAR	EQUIVALENT
Index Finger	Gyan Mudra	Jupiter	Knowledge
Middle Finger	Shuni Mudra	Saturn	Patience, wisdom, intelligence
Ring finger	Surya Mudra	Sun	Life energy, vitality
Pinky Finger	Buddhi Mudra	Mercury	Ability to communicate

✻ Following the pattern outlined below, chant in each of the three "speech forms of consciousness":
  • everyday life: normal or loud speech
  • being in love: whispering
  • mental plane: silent, only in your thoughts

Begin chanting at a normal volume for three minutes, then whisper for the next three minutes, followed by the pure internalization of sound for six minutes. Then whisper again for three minutes, and chant for the last three minutes at a normal volume. Afterward, inhale and exhale a few times.

* When thoughts uncontrollably come to the surface during the silent phase of your meditation, you should again start to whisper, chant loudly, then whisper again before coming back into silence. Do this as often as necessary.

* While repeating the mantra, imagine that the sound of each syllable is entering through the top of your head, the seventh chakra—the "gateway to the universe"—and then streaming out between your eyebrows from your third eye, the sixth chakra. This visualization of energy flow connects the disparate parts of the brain and cleanses the subconscious. The movement of your fingers and the pressure on your fingertips activates your meridian endpoints, facilitating energy flow to the brain.

* To conclude, stretch your arms up and out to the sides, lengthen your spine, and inhale and exhale deeply several times.

2. Using Meditation to Regulate an Irregular Menstrual Cycle

Many women have experienced irregular menstrual cycles since reaching the age of puberty. This doesn't necessarily mean they will suffer from fertility problems, just as a regular menstrual cycle is no guarantee of getting pregnant quickly. However, when hoping to get pregnant, it can be difficult to determine a woman's fertile period if her cycle fluctuates considerably from month to month. The following meditation, when practiced regularly, can help women regulate their menstrual cycles. The meditation facilitates letting go of negative thought patterns and promotes a fundamentally positive outlook on life. On the physical level, this breath meditation stimulates the pituitary and pineal glands, which both play an important role in maintaining emotional and physical health. Your bodily functions are significantly impacted by your endocrine glands, which regulate the hormones that keep you youthful, healthy, and emotionally stable.

The inhalation for this meditation is composed of four parts of the same length, and the exhalation follows in one breath. This meditation is traditionally used in yoga for general self-healing and for alleviating depression.

* Sit cross-legged or in a comfortable, upright position, and lay your hands on your knees, palms facing up.

* Inhale in four equal breaths—each one a short "sniffle"—and in so doing bring your thumb together with one finger at a time, as described during the Kirtan Kriya (see pages 119–120).

* Imagine "SA" while you bring your thumb and forefinger together, "TA" while bringing the thumb and middle finger together, "NA" with the thumb and ring finger, and "MA" with the thumb and pinky.

* With each "sniffle" pull your navel inward a bit more.

✳ Exhale in a single, extended breath. While exhaling, your hands should be lying in an open and relaxed manner on your knees, and your inner voice should be silent.

✳ Meditate this way for three minutes. Increase the time by one minute every day until you've reached seven minutes, and maintain this time for one week. If you'd like, continue to increase your meditation time incrementally by one minute each day, to a maximum of thirty-one minutes.

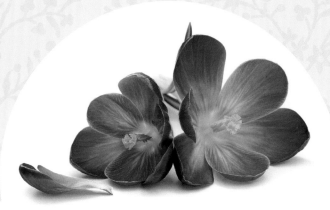

3. Meditation for Gratitude

"Be grateful? Why?" Perhaps this is what you ask yourself when seeing all of the women around you getting pregnant while you simply continue to be disappointed month after month. Each time it seems like your dream of having a baby is becoming ever more unattainable. As time goes on, you understandably start to lose your patience and composure even though you know that those states of mind play a part in creating the ideal conditions for getting pregnant. It's a vicious cycle—you fall into an increasingly agonized emotional state and become more fearful, even though you know doing so won't help you get pregnant. What should you do?

Approach the situation with dedication, gratitude, and positive thinking, and concentrate your awareness and attention on all that is good and beautiful in your life. Maybe it's a loving, supporting relationship, or good friends whom you know you can count on. Maybe you have a great job that you really enjoy, and enough money to lead a worry-free life. Or you have good health and a physically fit body. In everyone's life there are gifts to be found that should be valued. You can also feel gratitude for the challenges and difficulties you have encountered in your life, since they have helped you to grow and become the person you are today. Give yourself a gift and cultivate gratitude!

* Sit cross-legged for this meditation, and lay your hands fully relaxed upon your knees.
* Let your breath flow easily and naturally without trying to control it.
* The mantra for this meditation is *"Ek ong kar sat gur prasad—sat gur prasad ek ong kar."* This means, "Everything that happens is a blessing bestowed by the Creator. This insight has been given through grace." It is a mantra from the "Japji," the morning prayer of the Sikhs, and written in the scholarly language Gurmukhi, which is related to Sanskrit.
* Whisper this mantra or repeat it silently in your thoughts. Alternatively, you can chant along with a yoga CD.

✻ Imagine that you're being showered with blessings in the form of shooting stars falling from the heavens. Twinkling, brilliant stars are falling all around you, enveloping you in a cloak of stardust. Feel yourself blessed with the gifts of health, luck, well-being, and inner abundance. Take a moment to feel how all of these amazing gifts are being given to you, and how ready you are to receive them.

✻ Meditate with this in mind for five to eleven minutes.

✻ After concluding the recitation of your mantras, you will become aware of the blessings of your life. Look around you in gratitude at all of the blessings surrounding you.

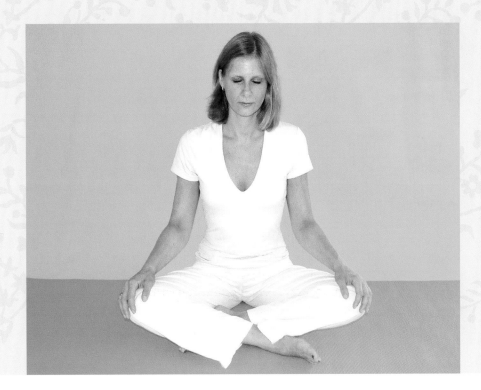

4. Practicing Mindfulness: Every Day Is a Gift

Start your day with practicing mindfulness. When you wake up in the morning give yourself the following blessing:

> Blessed are my hands that do so much for myself and others, and blessed are my feet that carry me so surely. Blessed is my head that thinks for me, and blessed is my heart that feels for me and beats so steadily. I bless my entire body in complete harmony.

Practice this daily for at least forty days. Doing so will generate a feeling of gratitude and deep inner satisfaction. Practicing mindfulness allows you to create an inner harmony that is independent of your external circumstances. Those who urgently yearn for children become emotionally dependent on the fulfillment of that wish, and can easily become unsatisfied and oversensitive. Giving yourself the gift of love, however, creates a harmonious force field in your heart. Inner harmony leads to a life filled with satisfaction and has the magnetic power to attract unending positivity to your life.

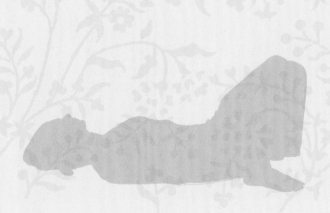

5. Breath Meditation for Emotional Balance

You can't exchange your body for another, but you can influence both the energy within your body and your state of mind and mood. When you feel tense and neurotic, you breathe primarily through your right nostril; when you feel sad or depressed, you breathe primarily through your left nostril. The left nostril is the end point for the primary energy channel known as *ida,* which runs along the length of the spine and is associated with the moon's energy—intuitive, emotional power. Breathing through the right nostril stimulates the primary energy canal known as *pingala,* which lies to the right of the spine and conducts the sun's energy—rational, action-oriented power.

The dominance of one nostril or the other usually alternates every two and a half hours, a phenomenon that the medical community discovered long before they were able to provide a scientific explanation for it. Yogis explain it as an energetic state that regulates and balances itself in a healthy organism. If you find that you have been stuck in the same mood or state of mind for a while, you can recover your emotional balance by consciously training yourself to breathe through alternating nostrils.

* Seat yourself in a comfortable meditation position, keeping your back straight.
* Close your eyes and relax your shoulders.
* Place your hands in the gyan mudra, with your thumb and index fingers touching, on your knees.
* Concentrate on the breath at the tip of your nose, and observe for three minutes which nostril you breathe through more often.
* When you believe you know which of your nostrils is dominant, concentrate on trying to alter your breathing pattern—simply through the power of your thoughts.
* If that proves too difficult a task, use your fingers to help you: Hold your active nostril closed with your thumb or forefinger.
* Practice for three minutes, increasing the time a bit each day until you reach eleven minutes.

CHAPTER 5

CONSCIOUS CONCEPTION THROUGH RELAXATION POSES AND VISUALIZATIONS

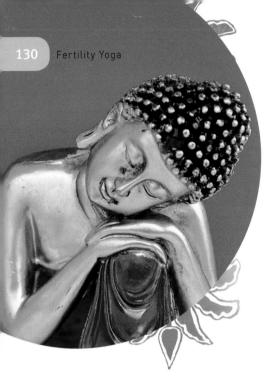

Reincarnation and the Principle of Karma

The yogic philosophy of reincarnation assumes that the soul of each child is attracted to its mother. It is said that children are the ones who seek out their parents, not the other way around. The baby's soul chooses a situation in which it can learn and grow. The power of attraction that enables a soul to choose a body is primarily influenced by the mental and spiritual state of the mother, but also by the father, the circumstances of the family, the environment, and the time.

This is called the principle of karma. The concept of karma is based on the Sanskrit word *karman* and means action or deed. It is a spiritual concept based on the idea that every action, every word, and every thought has a positive or negative consequence that won't necessarily occur immediately or even in this lifetime, but which will manifest in the next life. It is a principle of action and reaction. Karma doesn't result from any divine judgment, through mercy or punishment, but simply from the logical consequences of actions.

The doctrine of karma is associated with the cycle of rebirth and builds on the principle of cause and effect over several lifetimes. It is not only "bad" karma that leads to rebirth, but also "good" karma. According to the yogis once you no longer create any karma your soul escapes the cycle of rebirth and attains nirvana, the divine state of universal oneness.

Conscious Conception

The philosophy of yoga states that in the act of conception a woman opens her body and soul to permit another life to come into this world. In order to do so she must be in an extremely relaxed state, and sex with her partner should be loving and meditative. From a yogic perspective sex doesn't begin in the bedroom; it starts in the living room and simply continues in the bedroom. The foundation for conscious conception is a supportive, harmonious relationship in which both partners speak to each other often, meditate, and have an overall sense of well-being. Misunderstandings and disagreements should be resolved. There should be a readiness from both sides to communicate and find a balance between giving and taking. Trust, openness, and tenderness are prerequisites for conscious conception. Both should dedicate a significant amount of time to lovemaking, to melt into each other and enjoy the experience. If you speak German, you should also see my book *Erfüllter Sex mit Yoga* (Fulfilling Sex with Yoga).

The 120th Day

Many souls wait to reincarnate until they have had time to further develop and fulfill their destiny. Therefore, in the period immediately following conception, during the early stages of pregnancy, the soul that was attracted to the mother has not yet fully moved into the developing cells. There exists only a loose connection between body and soul, because Earth's magnetic field doesn't yet have any hold on the soul. Often a loose connection is established in this way with several souls, which sorts itself out as the pregnancy progresses.

Many women experience visions of their future child after conception or even some time before. When I was at the European Yoga Festival in 1996 and hadn't even begun to think about having a second child, I had a vivid dream of a baby. It occurred during the "oracle days" when I was alone in the forest. I dreamt of a sweet little blond boy named Elias. Exactly one year after the vision my son was born. According to the stars overhead at the time of his birth, he received a spiritual name that means "gift from the heavens." That he definitely is.

During the first four months after conception, it is also decided which soul will occupy the developing body. That means when the would-be mother works on her own development by inspiring positive changes within herself through the practice of fertility yoga, she will

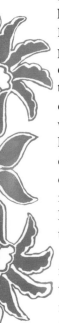

be better able to attract a soul that harmonizes with her character. Practicing yoga during pregnancy provides the developing child—in an especially intense way—with prana, the essential life energy usually obtained through breath, nutrition, water, light, and thoughts. It can also happen that the soul(s) hasn't yet decided who will incarnate in the developing body, which results in a miscarriage. That doesn't mean you have done anything wrong—something simply wasn't right at the time.

On the 120th day, the soul moves into the body. From this point forward the child is influenced by the mother, her vibrations transmitted to the baby and impressed upon his/her subconscious. For the duration of the pregnancy the child's karma can be improved if the mother acts selflessly and works on her spiritual development.

Relaxation Must Be Learned

Besides yoga and meditation practices, there is another important arena: conscious relaxation. Relaxation poses reduce emotional and mental stress and lead to a deep feeling of well-being in the here

and now. While in deep relaxation, the body activates its powers of self-healing, which work to balance the hormone system. It has been proven that women suffering from severe stress sometimes stop ovulating. The body "thinks" it is in danger, so it concentrates on its essential functions and activates its survival strategy, leaving no extra resources for "luxuries" such as reproduction. This negative effect can be exacerbated when a person creates additional emotional stress through her thoughts, for example by worrying about not getting pregnant after trying for such a long time despite "doing everything right," and finding no medical basis for her fertility issues. You can break this vicious cycle with yoga and conscious relaxation.

Relaxation is not a luxury that you can afford only when you have a lot of time or nothing better to do. It is a regular practice. Especially if you're a person who tends to tense up and hold all of your stress in your body instead of letting it simply flow through you, you need to practice relaxation. Just because you are more or less successful in getting a somewhat good night's sleep every night doesn't mean you are truly relaxing. Most men have a natural advantage in this realm, as many of them are able to turn off their stream of thoughts quite easily (exceptions exist, of course). Women, however, tend to take their problems and worries with them to bed, mulling them over again and again, even though they really yearn for relaxation, recovery, and distance. This causes nightmares and sleep disturbances.

Sleep is not the same thing as conscious, deep relaxation. For yogis, sleep represents a state of unconsciousness, while a state of deep mental and physical relaxation is located in the precarious balance between waking and sleeping. In this *nidra* state, patterns of tension and stress are resolved, which can be demonstrated with the help of an EEG machine. The brain finds itself in a state of light relaxation, transmitting alpha waves and, with continued practice, theta waves that can be measured in meditation and deeper relaxation. Some yogis are even able to consciously transport themselves into a delta state of trance or deep sleep within a short span of time.

Those who regularly practice deep relaxation lower their stress levels, promote restful sleep, and reactivate their natural fertility.

"The Mind Is Like a Monkey Sitting at the Wheel"

All relaxation poses are on the one hand about letting go of your body, and on the other about relaxing your thoughts. Observe your thoughts from a neutral perspective. Simply let them come and go, and don't hold on to them. This can be difficult at the beginning if you tend to entangle yourself in your patterns of thought because you identify with your mind, your ego. Instead of relaxing you are perhaps lying uncomfortably on the floor, unable to stop the thoughts that are only making you feel worse. As the yogis say, "The mind is like a monkey sitting at the wheel."

Imagine that you are planning to take a trip by hired car, and you have a clear plan laid out. You have determined your route and filled the gas tank. You have packed supplies and are well rested and in good spirits. When you get into the car the driver speeds off immediately.

Everything goes well at first, but then you notice that he's driving like a maniac, crossing over the median dividers, narrowly avoiding accidents, and then driving along calmly again as if nothing had happened. You realize that instead of the driver you hired, a monkey is sitting at the wheel! Even though he has mastered the technicalities of driving, he ignores all of your instructions and requests, takes detours, and simply stops at will to take catnaps. In short, he does what he wants, not what you want. Would you tolerate a driver like that? No—you would throw him out of the car at the first opportunity.

Our mind sometimes works in a similar way. We think we have it under control. We believe that our mind serves us; even more commonly we believe that our mind *is* us. We falsely identify with the monkey behind the wheel. We believe that our thoughts and feelings constitute our being and form the essence of our identity. In fact, the opposite is really the case.

Your mind in most cases does what *it* wants to, pulling you into dangerous mental whirlpools and grueling thought patterns, such as why, when everyone else is having children left and right, you are having difficulties, what you must be doing wrong, how you should change, etc. You lie sleepless in bed, tossing and turning while developing feelings of guilt or resentment toward your partner, your doctors, and yourself—not to mention feeling horribly unhappy and depressed. And all of this happens just because you trusted the monkey sitting at the wheel.

Yogis have a saying: "Don't believe everything you think." The first step is recognizing that you are not your mind or your thoughts; you have an essential core of being that remains uninfluenced by your mind's empty chatter and incessant attempts to explain the world to you. This core is called "SAT NAM," the true identity; it is of this that you are truly made.

Taming the monkey, or restraining your mind, is the true goal of yoga. When you succeed in quieting the unending ramblings of your mind for even a moment, you have caught a glimpse of what in yoga is called *shunia,* or the void. And this void, this silence, is so exquisite that once you have experienced it you always want more.

To accomplish this you must inwardly take a step back in order to observe your thoughts from a neutral point of view. Maintain some distance from yourself, like an independent observer. Then give your mind something easy but constant to do: imagine the mantra

"SAAAT" while inhaling, and "NAAAM" while exhaling. Do this again and again. Feed the monkey. If that mantra is too easy and your mind continues to produce thoughts in the background, try another, for example the Mul mantra in table below. In the left column is the mantra to hold in your mind; in the right column is the translation.

The legend behind this mantra is that Nanak, one of the ten Sikh gurus, is said to have spoken it after awakening enlightened from a three-day underwater meditative trance.

EK	One
ONG	is the cosmic vibration
KAR	with creation.
SAT NAM	This is also my true essence.
KARTA PURAKH	Everything was created
NIRBHAU NIRVAIR	without fear, without anger,
AKAL MURAT AJUNI	without death or birth,
SAIBHANG	emerging luminous from itself.
GURPARSAD JAP	This realization is the gift of meditation.
AD SACH	It is the original truth,
JUGAD SACH	the truth of all ages,
HAI BHI SACH	the truth now,
NANAK HOSI BHI SACH	and, Nanak, it will always be the truth.

Repeat the mantra silently to yourself, and in so doing liberate yourself from the yoke of your unwanted thoughts.

Relaxation Poses

Relax daily in one of the following poses for at least eleven to twenty minutes. For a woman to tap into her intuitive powers she should relax in this or another way at least once per day, and even better twice per day. Only when a woman is relaxed is she at her most intuitive and strong-nerved, which allows her to live out her highest potential and be both a good partner and mother. This has been said since the time of the ancient yogis.

"Dear, I have to relax. I'm doing it for us." Is there a better argument for taking some time daily to relax?

1. Relaxing in the Corpse Pose

❋ Lie down on your back on your yoga mat, a carpet, or a blanket. The room should be pleasantly warm and well-ventilated. Cover yourself with a light blanket or sheet. Stretch out your legs and position your feet about three feet apart, in order to properly relax your back and pelvis. Feel how the sheet covering you rises and falls with your breath.

❋ Place your hands on your abdomen and shift your attention to them. Carefully direct your breath to your uterus and pelvic organs. Lift your stomach upon inhaling, and let it fall back down upon exhaling. Let your breath flow in and out in its own natural rhythm. Don't try to control it; simply trust its rhythm.

❋ Feel the earth's gravitational pull upon your body. Let it carry you. The earth is supporting you—accept this, and feel all of your tension melting away.

❋ Maybe you'd like to listen to some soft, relaxing music that would help you better zone out. Or imagine your thoughts floating by like clouds in the sky. Whenever a thought arises take a moment to observe it, and then release it upon your next breath.

❋ This is not the time to take a nap. Try instead to balance on the threshold between waking and sleeping, even when it might seem tempting to fall asleep.

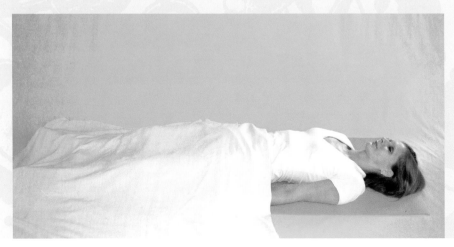

2. Relaxing in the Stomach Pose

✳ Lie on your stomach. Whatever you're lying on should be soft enough that it doesn't give you back pain. Either turn your head to the side or fold your hands under your forehead to form a kind of pillow. Spread your legs slightly apart, letting your heels fall outward, your toes touching. Establish contact with the earth.

✳ Feel where your body touches the ground, and where there are air pockets between your body and the earth. Breathe consciously into your stomach and feel how your stomach presses against the ground. Send your breath into your back and shoulders, and feel yourself relaxing more and more deeply.

✳ Listening to some nice, relaxing music will facilitate your ability to let go.

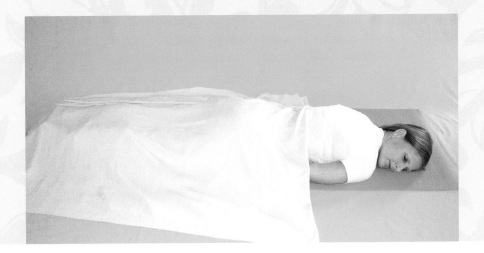

3. Relaxing in the Gurpranam Pose

✳ Place one or two blankets beside you and sit up on your heels. If this is uncomfortable, place a folded blanket behind your knees or sit on a meditation cushion. Have meditation music playing softly in the background.

✳ While leaning forward, pull one blanket up over your back. Bend down until your forehead touches the floor, and fully extend your arms forward, stretching them as far as you can, your palms touching.

✳ This position has a simultaneous relaxing and stimulating effect upon the female reproductive organs. It also relaxes and strengthens your nervous system. If you sense any unpleasant pressure, open your knees a bit so that your upper thighs press less on your stomach.

✳ As you inhale imagine your breath originating at the base of your spine and pouring upward out of your crown chakra, and then on exhaling imagine it flowing back down to your lower back.

✳ Hold this position for several minutes and observe the flow of your breath. To conclude, push yourself up with your hands until you are sitting upright. Be careful, as you might feel a bit dizzy.

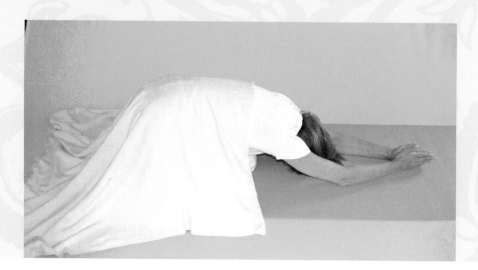

4. Relaxing in the Child's Pose

✷ Sit on your heels and bend forward until your forehead is resting on the floor. Stretch your arms backward, placing your hands next to your heels on the floor. Your palms should be facing up, and your fingers relaxed and slightly curved. Make yourself small and round. Your knees can be either open or closed.

✷ Listen to your own breath and/or relaxing music, and for a few minutes simply let everything go.

✷ This relaxing position is particularly good for your back.

Women should regularly practice a visualization with the aim of building a loving relationship with their uterus, the future home of their child. Imagine that you're in a relaxed position, that your child wants to come to you just as much as you want it, that it is being born. Envision your special relationship with one another, and tell yourself that your current wait is simply an extension of your future pregnancy. It doesn't matter if your child needs a little more time to arrive; in fact, it's a positive thing that you have some time to prepare.

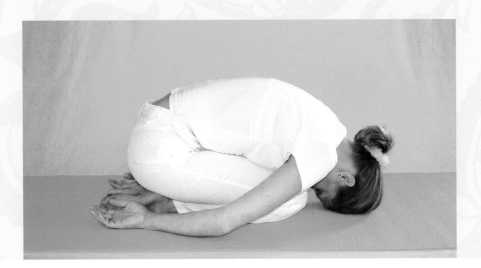

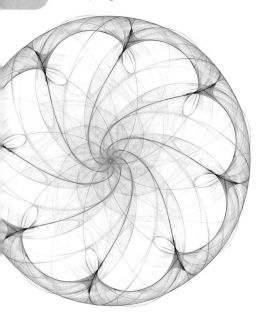

Visualizing Your Desire to Have a Child

Dream travel and visualizations aid in fulfilling your desire for children. Whatever moves us inwardly has outward effects, and vice versa.

The events of your day enter into your nightly dreams and are processed there. We also perceive the outer world through the filter of our inner perspective and attitude. We create our own reality through the ways in which we perceive it. There is no objective truth because everyone sees the world through their own subjective lens.

Consciously planned dream travel offers the possibility to explore and create your inner world. It can help you to find new ways to negotiate a reality that you otherwise experience negatively, and to reinterpret events, both past and present. Toni Cade Bambara, a famous African-American feminist, once said, "Revolution begins with the self, in the self."

The following dream-travel sequence will stimulate the flow of energy into your chakras, the energy centers of the body. Chakras, as described earlier, are psycho-energetic centers, each a rotating vortex of energy in the psychic and physical bodies. Engaging in this visualization will have a harmonizing effect on your vital functions and on your endocrine system.

The dream-travel sequence is best undertaken with the guidance of another person, one whom you like and trust and who will read it aloud to you. It can be read by a trusted friend or partner, or you can record yourself reading it and then play it back for the journey.

Set aside approximately twenty minutes of undisturbed time. If you'd like, put on some soft, relaxing music in the background.

1. Dream Travel Through Your Chakras

Lie down comfortably on your yoga mat, a carpet, or a mattress. Your body should be in the corpse pose described earlier. Feel free to put a small pillow under your head if you'd like. Cover yourself so that you won't get cold. Position your legs slightly apart so that your thighs don't touch. Your feet should fall open. Your arms are placed along your sides, palms up and fingers curved slightly inward. Close your eyes and keep them closed until the end of the exercise.

Be aware of your entire body. Perceive the points where it touches the floor and the gaps of air between it and the earth. Feel how certain body parts touch the floor: your heels, your calves, the backs of your thighs, your buttocks, parts of your back, your shoulder blades, the backs of your arms, your hands. Feel how your neck and the back of your head touch the floor.

Let go. Let the weight of your body sink into the ground. The earth is holding you. Let it support you. Feel how, with every breath, you release more and more of the tension you have been holding in your body, and let yourself sink lower and lower into the earth.

Take a deep breath, and upon exhaling release all of your physical tension. Inhale deeply again, and upon exhaling release all of your mental tension. Inhale deeply for a third time, and upon exhaling let go of all of your emotional tension.

Now let go of your breath. Become aware of how your navel rises and falls with your breath. Don't try to control your breath, but simply observe its natural rhythm.

Relax. Let everything go. Your body will relax all by itself while you trace your awareness throughout your body, each part at a time. Form a mental image of each body part and repeat its name silently.

Bring your awareness to your feet: your toes, heels, the soles of your feet, your ankles. Now shift your awareness to your buttocks, pelvis, hips, and lower torso. Focus your attention on your stomach, chest, ribs, and breasts. Next move your awareness to the back side of your body and feel the left side of your back. Feel the right side of your back. Feel your spine, each vertebra at a time, starting with your tailbone on up to your head. Feel your shoulder blades, shoulders, upper arms, elbows, lower arms, hands, and each individual finger. Shift your awareness to your neck, throat, and face. Feel your jaw, mouth, nose, cheeks, ears, and forehead. Feel your scalp, your head, your whole body, your whole body, your whole body.

Be totally present within yourself. Feel safe and one with the universe. Visualize your body in your mind's eye; observe how it is lying calmly, comfortably, and completely relaxed on the floor.

Now shift your awareness to your spine, to its twenty-six vertebrae strung like pearls on a necklace. Feel your spine and travel to its base. There you observe a flower in bloom, covered in drops of dew and framed by beautiful green leaves. Here lies your root chakra, muladhara. This chakra is red; imagine a red lotus blossom with four petals. Muladhara is your anchor, your solid grounding in the world, the foundation of your stability and inner strength. Now move a bit higher to the second chakra, swadhisthana, located between your pubic bone and navel. Here you observe an orange lotus blossom with six petals. Swadhisthana signifies joy, lust for life, sensuality, and the power of creation and reproduction. Procreation and conception are grounded

here. Next observe manipura, your third chakra, which lies behind your navel. It is a lotus blossom with ten golden petals. Manipura signifies self-confidence, vigor, and courage. Travel up your spine a bit higher and observe anahata, the heart chakra, which lies behind your heart. Anahata is a lotus blossom with twelve green or pink petals, and symbolizes love, compassion, and healing. Go a little higher, up to your throat, and observe vishuddha, your throat chakra. It is a lotus blossom with sixteen blue petals, and signifies truth, communication, and speech. The next chakra is ajna, your third eye, located between your eyebrows. Ajna has only two midnight-blue petals and signifies intuition, foresight, and holistic thought. Finally, move up to the crown of your head. Here lies the seventh chakra, sahasrara, your crown chakra. Observe a thousand-petalled lotus blossom with sparkling white petals, your connection to the cosmos, the gateway to the universe, wholeness, and bliss.

Shift your awareness once again to ajna…to vishuddha…to anahata… to manipura…to swadhisthana… to muladhara. When the light of the moon falls upon you, the petals of these lotus blossoms sparkle like diamonds. Some are simple, others glowing, shimmering like gold and silver, like diamonds and stars. Feel the energetic vibrations of your chakras, and with your breath carry prana, the cleansing and harmonizing life energy, to all of your chakras. Imagine upon exhaling that you are giving up everything you no longer need, and upon inhaling that you are free and open to the new.

Observe again your first chakra, between the anus and urethra; your second chakra, at the top of your pubic bone; your third chakra, at your navel; your fourth chakra, behind your heart; your fifth chakra, at your throat; your sixth chakra, between your eyebrows; and your seventh chakra, at the crown of your head. Feel how each chakra affects you, which feelings and sensations they bring up. Observe your true nature and acknowledge your tasks, your opportunities for growth. Accept yourself with great love, compassion, and forgiveness. Bless yourself. Let joy shine onto your life and your world. Feel yourself enveloped in a protective, healing light.

(The reader should pause for several minutes.)

Now start to come slowly back. Bid farewell to your visualizations and dreams. Inhale and exhale again, more deeply and forcefully, and begin to wiggle your fingers and toes. Draw circles with your hands and feet in the air, and stretch out. Stretch your arms above your head and elongate your body. Bend your knees with feet flat on the floor, and let your knees fall first to the left and then to the right. Draw your knees to your chest, wrapping your arms around them, and roll gently back and forth on your spine. Now come into a sitting position.

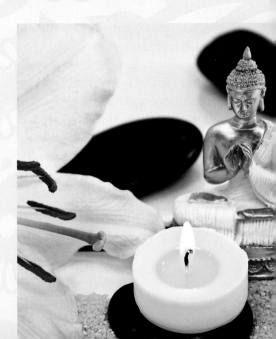

2. Visualization for Ovarian Follicle Development and Egg Implantation

"Just let it go." "Relax and it will happen." "There is no medical reason why it shouldn't work." "From a medical standpoint there is nothing else we can do." "Don't dwell on it, simply let it happen."

All of these are well-intentioned pieces of advice that are often given to couples trying to have children, but they don't help. How can you simply relax and "let it happen" when your wish for a child is so overwhelming that it affects other areas of your life? You can't simply stop thinking about it, but you *can* try to influence your thinking—to train the monkey—by creating positive images in your mind that in turn make you feel good and thereby stimulate your hormones. The body reacts to emotional signals, to unconscious vibrations. When women want to convince their bodies to become pregnant, it's important to send the right signals and images from the unconscious. Know that the unconscious doesn't recognize negation; when you say, for example, that you shouldn't think about pink elephants the first thing your

unconscious mind will produce is an image of pink elephants. If you'd like to have a dialogue with your unconscious, you must communicate in positive images that will immediately and directly reach it, without taking a detour through your critical mind.

Women trying to conceive can make use of visualization as a helpful tool. Use the power of your imagination to create a positive image that will redirect the energy of your thoughts. Try creating a positive image of your ovaries in your mind. It doesn't have to be anatomically correct. Simply create an image that you like, perhaps that of two fruit trees. Every day you observe how the ripening process is coming along, how the buds are growing into fruit ever larger and riper. Choose an image for yourself, perhaps that of a garden, perhaps an impressionistic painting of your belly that is painted more each day, anything that allows you to observe the process of growth and maturation. The only important thing is that you find the image pleasant, that it moves you. Turn your awareness inward daily and shift your attention to the image of your ovaries, with you as a well-wisher observing their activities.

It is important not to pressure your body into producing high-quality, "turbo" eggs at light speed. Simply observe your eggs developing with calmness and serenity, from the viewpoint of your true self.

After ovulation, alter your visualization a bit: Perhaps imagine your uterus as a pleasantly lit, comfortable red cave or a comfy nest—or however you'd like to visualize it. Observe your uterus becoming ever warmer, softer, and more inviting, and a small, fertilized egg nestling inside it, feeling safe, secure, and well provided for in its new home. Maintain this image as long as you'd like. Visualization practice helps ease the impatience and anxiety that have built up through the endless waiting for pregnancy. Instead of feeling helpless week after week, utilize the power of positive images to support yourself. The power of auto-suggestion has been scientifically proven; studies have shown that it leads to increased circulation in the uterus and ovaries through their relaxation and expansion.

Making sure to always eat healthy, constantly taking precautions to behave in a fertility-supportive manner, and/or practicing yoga can be exhausting and unenjoyable over the long term. As you partake of all the useful alternative therapies, practice good nutrition, follow the behavioral recommendations, and don't neglect sensual enjoyment! A child is a product of love celebrated between two partners, of the tenderness and pleasure through which you express your sexuality as man and woman. There are other aspects of life that can have positive effects on your fertility and simultaneously produce a high enjoyment factor. That is the topic of the next chapter.

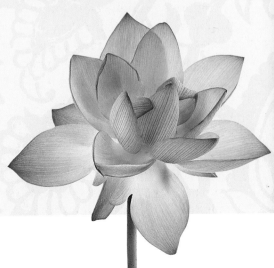

CHAPTER 6

ENJOYING ALL
OF YOUR SENSES

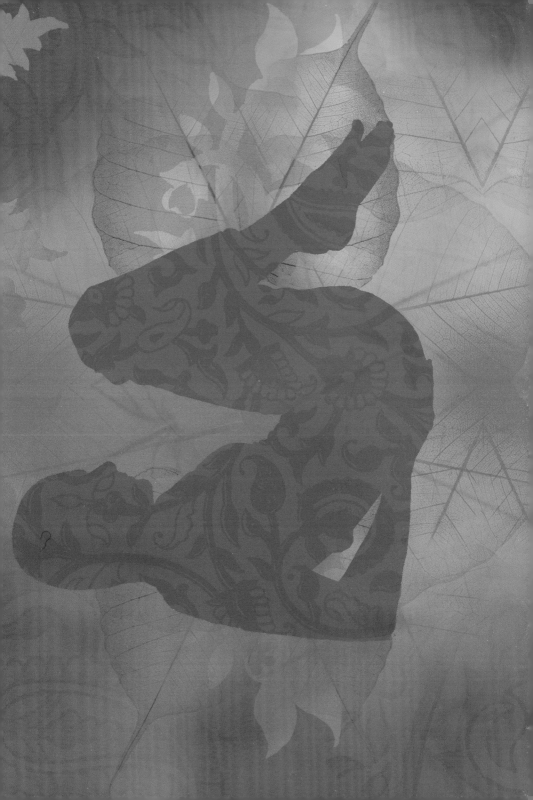

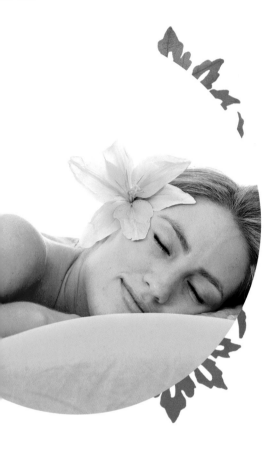

The Sunny Side of Life

There have been so many reports in recent years of the harmful effects the sun can have on the skin that people have almost forgotten the positive effects the sun can have on the mind, mood, and hormones. The natural light of the sun has an antidepressant effect—and as we already know depression hinders fertility. Moreover, the epiphysis or pineal gland serves as the body's "light meter." According to the yogic tradition it is the location of the seventh chakra, the "gateway to the universe." The pineal gland is an important part of the body's system for controlling reproductive hormones. If it doesn't get enough sunlight this system can't work properly. Studies have shown that one hour a day of sunlight is optimal for increased fertility. This doesn't mean the sun actually has to be shining; you can get your daily intake of sunlight on a cloudy day.

Each section in this chapter describes a way of increasing the sensual potential of your everyday life. Think of the chapter as a banquet of offerings, and pick and choose the ones that most appeal to you.

Belly Dance

Many think that belly dance was developed in order to seduce men. What is today often considered a tourist attraction or a social love ritual was in earlier eras danced mostly in secret, with men not allowed to watch. Belly dancing is based on ancient fertility rites, its movements aimed at strengthening the diaphragm and stomach muscles, which are used during sex, pregnancy, and birth.

When women practice belly dance while trying to conceive, it doesn't mean they will become mystically pregnant. Instead, they will become conscious of the ancient power of the feminine and their own sensuality and creative energy, all the while strengthening their deep musculature. Belly dancing stimulates ovulation and heightens sexual feeling. To learn belly dance, it is best to take a class. There are also other traditions of fertility dance, many with African origins.

Erotic Partner Dance

Have you ever heard the saying that a person should dance with their partner before marrying them? Dancing often reveals far more about a person than deep conversation. Connecting on this physical-sensual level is often more powerful than connection based on the rational mind and life plans. Dancing with your partner is an enjoyable experience, strengthens the second chakra, and can stimulate fertility. Dancing stimulates blood flow to the reproductive areas of the body, making conception more likely.

Even if it doesn't lead to an immediate pregnancy, take a dance class with your partner. Argentinean tango is a great option. Because it is the vertical expression of horizontal emotions, it is the most sensual of dances, and it can permanently eroticize your relationship and increase your capacity for shared vibration with your partner. In Argentinean tango you dance in a permanent, tight embrace. The point is not to learn complicated combinations but to learn how to move together to the music, to feel each other, to heighten your awareness of each other's body. In that sense dance isn't too different from yoga. Getting into the dance flow with your partner can be a highly meditative experience. Partner dance directly affects the right side of the brain, stimulating emotions, intuition, and relaxation. It also solidifies your connection to your partner and creates a stable, lasting foundation for the upcoming, nerve-racking years of parenthood.

Sex as Fun, Not a Chore

At first it's a titillating, sexy prospect: you finally don't have to worry about birth control, can have unprotected sex whenever you want, and can give your passion free reign. This is the way it usually begins when a couple decides to have a child. The thought that it could happen "right now" is always present when they have sex, and it functions as an aphrodisiac. But when month after month passes with no pregnancy, the mood can flip in the other direction. Having sex changes from being fun into an obligation that becomes more and more routine, with the goal of finally getting pregnant. Passion is gradually given a secondary role until it disappears into the background altogether.

What first began as a loving wish starts to frustrate and exhaust you because your plans aren't coming into fulfillment as fast as you had expected. You eventually have sex only during your most fertile days, when sperm are in their prime and the egg is mature. Perhaps both partners feel like they have been reduced to their sexual functions: the man as a sperm donor under procreative pressure and the woman as a baby-making machine. If you have reached this point, pull the emergency brake—don't wait a single minute longer.

Remember when you were both young and in love, or newly married? You couldn't keep your hands off each other. You made love often and enthusiastically, and exactly as you wanted, not in positions meant to maximize conception.

Try to place more of your trust in Mother Nature, and you will find your way. Think back on the uncomplicated early stages of being in love, and only have sex when you both crave each other—even if that means you might lose a week of "precious time."

Sexual Positions

People used to believe that the missionary position was the best position for successful conception. After the man ejaculated the woman was supposed to hold her pelvis up, not moving for at least a half hour. Today there are better understandings of conception. Every sexual position in which the man ejaculates deep into the woman's vagina is good. You don't have to raise your legs afterwards so that the sperm will find their way to your egg. Some women fear that gravity has a negative effect on fertilization, but sperm are fast swimmers and will find their way to the egg if they are meant to. Come together again, with no pressure this time, and see where your passion leads you. Play with each other, and try out new positions, places, techniques.

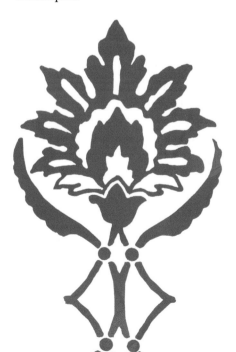

New underwear or lingerie can work wonders, making you feel seductive and sexy. Try role playing, let yourself be tied up, book a romantic getaway to surprise your partner, watch pornographic films together—anything that adds variety and gets you out of your routine.

Stress-Relieving Massage

When sex increasingly becomes something you have to do, rather than something you want to do, it starts to become stressful. Mutual massage can be a relaxing way to initiate an erotic encounter. Massage lowers the body's levels of the stress hormone cortisol and increases brain levels of the neurotransmitters serotonin and dopamine. Both of these hormones make you feel good and increase your receptiveness to connecting with others. They are usually released into the body when you experience joy. After extensively massaging one another sensually, you will probably feel like having sex—and even if you don't, you just did something wonderful for each other.

Giving Up Lubricants and Oral Sex

When it comes to conception, there are unfortunately certain things that you have to temporarily give up. A study from Belfast, Ireland, showed that saliva significantly decreases the mobility of sperm, by 50 percent during the first five minutes of sexual intercourse and by 95 percent during the following fifteen min-utes. It could therefore be best for both sides to hold off on oral sex—at least during your most fertile period.

Oil-based lubricants should also be avoided when you're trying to conceive, because they can kill sperm. Fragrances and synthetic flavorings can do the same. Lubricants also decrease the mobility of surviving sperm. There are natural alternatives that are safe, such as olive oil, canola oil, or egg whites. Some nonspermicidal lubricants are safe as well. It is best, however,

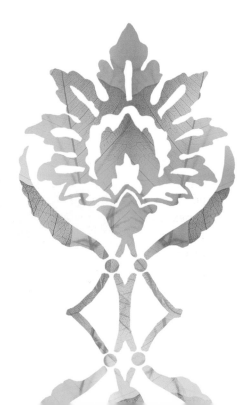

to simply enjoy enough foreplay so that you produce more than enough of your own natural lubrication.

Pleasant Afternoon Sex

Having sex in the afternoon is recommended both because you won't be as tired as you are in the evening or at night, and because the time of day actually increases your probability of getting pregnant, as shown in a study done in Italy. According to the study men produced more and faster sperm in the afternoon than at any other time of day. Here's a recommendation for an enjoyable weekend for two: Go out to eat on Friday evening, go out dancing late into the night—preferably Argentinean tango—and sleep in on Saturday morning. Have an extensive, luxurious breakfast, and spend the afternoon in bed playing erotic games. Then repeat the schedule that night and the next day. This period is a wonderful time in your life. Enjoy it together using all of your senses, before this interval of calm and tranquility is gone.

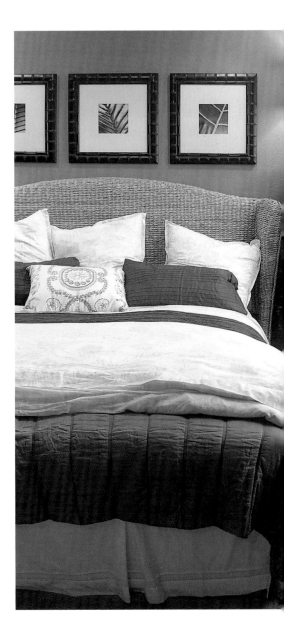

Afterword: When Nothing Helps

Perhaps you've reached the point where you have tried everything, including medical fertility treatment. You still really want children, but are no longer sure how to make it happen or if it is even possible. In this case, the only thing that helps is *letting go.*

You shouldn't renounce your desire for children, but you should stop everything that you are doing to try to make this desire a reality, both inwardly and outwardly, actively or passively. If you are charting your temperature, throw the chart out. Get rid of all of your fertility and nutrition books. Make love with your partner only when you want to, and do it for yourselves, not with the goal of getting pregnant. Don't stop talking with your partner, however. Express your feelings, including the painful ones; don't sweep them under the rug.

Put a stop to all of the questions from well-meaning outsiders, and make it clear that you don't want to talk about the subject anymore. Take care of yourself and do good things for yourself. Have fun, relax, continue practicing yoga, start a new hobby, or take a trip to a place you've never been. Trust the wisdom of your body, even when it doesn't seem to be doing what you want it to.

There may come a point when you will have to let go of your hopes for having children. It can be a long, difficult mourning process, and one through which you may need professional help. But in life we must all walk the path of letting go and saying goodbye, whether or not we have children.

Recommended Reading

Glenville, Marilyn. *Boost Your Fertility: New Solutions for Conceiving Quickly and Having a Healthy Pregnancy as Soon as Possible.* Beverly, MA: Fair Winds Press, 2009.

Jones, Carol Fulwiler. *Managing the Stress of Infertility: How to Balance Your Emotions, Get the Support You Need, and Deal with Painful Social Situations When You're Trying to Become Pregnant.* Atlanta, GA: Fraser Davis Press, 2012.

Lauersen, Niels H., and Colette Bouchez. *Green Fertility: Nature's Secrets for Making Babies: A Powerful Proven Plan to Help You Get Pregnant Fast & Have a Healthy Baby.* Princeton, NJ: Ivy League Press, 2010.

Lewis, Randine. *The Infertility Cure: The Ancient Chinese Wellness Program for Getting Pregnant and Having Healthy Babies.* New York: Little, Brown and Company, 2005.

McQuaid, Matthew. *A Spiritual Path to Overcoming Infertility: Creating Your Miracle Family Now.* Lakeport, CA: Reverence Press, 2006.

Petigara, Jill, and Lynn Jensen. *Yoga and Fertility: A Journey to Health and Healing.* New York: Demos Health, 2012.

Quinn, Tami. *The Infertility Cleanse: Detox, Diet and Dharma for Fertility.* Forres, Scotland: Findhorn Press, 2011.

Sivananda Yoga Vedanta Centers. *The Yoga Cookbook: Vegetarian Food for Body and Mind.* New York: Touchstone, 1999.

Sharon, Gannon. *Yoga and Vegetarianism: The Diet of Enlightenment.* San Rafael, CA: Mandala Publishing, 2008.

Weschler, Toni. *Taking Charge of Your Fertility: The Definitive Guide to Natural Birth Control, Pregancy Achievement, and Reproductive Health.* New York: First Quill, 2006.

Related Books from Hunter House Publishers

Cavallucci, Danielle, and Yvonne Fulbright. *Your Orgasmic Pregnancy.* Alameda, CA: Hunter House Publishers, 2008.

Kass-Annese, Barbara, and Hal Danzer. *Natural Birth Control Made Simple.* Alameda, CA: Hunter House Publishers, 2003. Also available in Spanish with the title *Simples Métodos de Control de la Natalidad.*

Raab, Diana M. *Getting Pregnant and Staying Pregnant*, 3rd edition. Alameda, CA: Hunter House Publishers, 1999.

Raab, Diana M., with Errol Norwitz. *Your High-Risk Pregnancy: A Practical and Supportive Guide.* Alameda, CA: Hunter House Publishers, 2009.

Röst, Cecile. *Relieving Pelvic Pain During and After Pregnancy.* Alameda, CA: Hunter House Publishers, 2007.

Index